"Rich with practical information, *The Pregnancy and Postpartum Mood Workbook*
accessible for even the most exhausted or distressed parent or partner. This in
can be used independently or as a companion to psychotherapy. Warren and Berger have created an
essential tool that's long been missing in the toolbox for family well-being. Many thanks to you both
for the support and assistance this book will provide!"

**Pec Indman, PA, EdD, MFT, PMH-C**, *co-author of* Beyond the Blues:
A Guide to Understanding and Treating Prenatal and Postpartum Depression

"The thoughtfulness and expertise in this workbook is unmatched. By combining necessary information
and very usable skills in an easily accessible format, it will feel like having both brilliant psychotherapists
right by your side. This is an essential addition to the much-needed resources for any pregnant or
postpartum person, as well as for the clinicians who support them."

**Katayune Kaeni, Psy.D., PMH-C**, *Mom & Mind podcast;*
*Postpartum Support International executive board member-at-large*

"This is an 'Everything I needed to know about perinatal mood and anxiety disorders (PMADS)' guided
self-help workbook for any woman who is pregnant, postpartum or wanting to learn more about
PMADs. This workbook is also a wonderful tool for maternal mental health practitioners to use with
their clients. With attention to special populations, it is inclusive and accessible to all women. It provides mothers the knowledge to better understand their affliction so they can start battling it success-
fully. It teaches women skills, so they not only survive their emotions when having a baby but thrive."

**Alison Reminick, M.D.**, *associate professor of psychiatry; director, Women's*
*Reproductive Mental Health Program, University of California, San Diego, USA*

"Although there are many wonderful books about postpartum depression, Bethany Warren and
Dr. Berger have provided readers with the most comprehensive and current workbook on the market on
how to manage struggles with pregnancy and postpartum mood disruptions. Their voices are relatable,
their knowledge is vast, and they succeed in reminding the reader that they are not alone and can get
better with the skills provided in this workbook."

**Maria Henke Elswick, M.D., OB/GYN**, *maternal mental health specialist*

"They nailed it. The impact of pregnancy and postpartum on emotions should not be overlooked and
emphasis on mental health is paramount in recovery during the 4th trimester. Beyond addressing
Postpartum Depression, Bethany and Beth help new parents navigate this difficult time by addressing
important topics such as the entire range of mood symptoms a new parent might experience, how
to interweave self-care in a feasible way, and the impact that having a baby and having depression,
anxiety, and other mood struggles can have on a relationship. They make this workbook user friendly
for hard working/sleep deprived new parents."

**Jay M. Goldberg, M.D., Ob/Gyn**

"This is the book we've all been waiting for. Warren and Berger use their expertise to create the ultimate
go-to bible on mental healing during pregnancy and beyond. Effortlessly, and with a warm and friendly
style, they hew a mountain of research-informed methods into practical bite-sized chunks proven to
help women on their path into motherhood. No mother or (maternal health therapist!) can afford to
miss this valuable resource."

**Dr. Sarah Simmons**, *Psychiatrist*

# THE PREGNANCY AND POSTPARTUM MOOD WORKBOOK

This book helps you throughout your pregnancy and postpartum/postnatal recovery. By helping you understand what you are feeling, and teaching you empirically validated new skills so you can manage your changing moods, you can work toward feeling better.

Becoming a new parent is one of the biggest changes one can face in life. You are experiencing enormous changes biologically, hormonally, and emotionally. Your whole life may seem uprooted. It makes sense that you might be feeling significant mood changes as well. With one out of five mothers and one out of ten partners experiencing depression and anxiety when having a baby, this workbook will remind you that you are not alone.

This workbook is written with sleep-deprived new parents in mind, providing helpful information in short, digestible segments. These are intermixed with thought-provoking activities such as brief journaling prompts and suggestions for tangible steps to make small, realistic changes. You can pick it up and put it down, reading it on your timing, without the information becoming overwhelming. The workbook covers the entire range of mood symptoms, from the Baby Blues, to anxiety, depression, bipolar disorder, PTSD, OCD, and more.

*The Pregnancy and Postpartum Mood Workbook* uses inclusive language and content applicable to all new parents. There are chapters uniquely dedicated to building attachment, managing awful thoughts, bringing awareness to your partner's mental health, parenting babies in the NICU or with medical issues, and exploring culture, identity, and mental health. There is also a resource section with a wide array of support available to meet the needs of any parent. Adoptive and single parents, LGBTQ+ and heterosexual parents, as well as clinicians and birth workers will find this book to be an invaluable resource.

**Bethany Warren, LCSW, PMH-C**, is an experienced psychotherapist certified in both EMDR therapy and Perinatal Mental Health. She regularly provides trainings and lectures on women's mental health and trauma.

**Beth Creager Berger, Ph.D.**, is a psychologist with over twenty years of experience specializing in anxiety disorders and Perinatal Mental Health. She frequently lectures to physicians and community groups about PMADs.

# THE PREGNANCY AND POSTPARTUM MOOD WORKBOOK

## The Guide to Surviving Your Emotions When Having a Baby

Bethany Warren, LCSW, PMH-C and Beth Creager Berger, Ph.D.

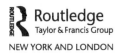
Routledge
Taylor & Francis Group

NEW YORK AND LONDON

First published 2022
by Routledge
605 Third Avenue, New York, NY 10158

and by Routledge
2 Park Square, Milton Park, Abingdon, Oxon, OX14 4RN

*Routledge is an imprint of the Taylor & Francis Group, an informa business*

*Library of Congress Cataloging-in-Publication Data*
A catalog record for this book has been requested

ISBN: 978-0-367-69965-9 (hbk)
ISBN: 978-0-367-69966-6 (pbk)
ISBN: 978-1-003-14402-1 (ebk)

DOI: 10.4324/9781003144021

Typeset in Stone Serif
by Apex CoVantage, LLC

Dedicated to all of the parents struggling through the darkness until you can again find the light

# CONTENTS

# ACKNOWLEDGMENTS

Throughout the workbook we talk about the importance of the village to raise a child and support parents. In truth, it took a village to create our workbook as well. We would like to thank everyone who inspired and supported us in the writing of this workbook.

A profound thank you to all of our clients who we have seen throughout our careers. You inspire us with your bravery of showing up, doing hard things and by being vulnerable in our work together. It's such a privilege to watch you change and grow and heal. You're the ultimate reason we wrote this workbook.

Thank you to our parents and families, and particularly our supportive husbands for all of your patience and encouragement throughout the years of us writing our workbook. We couldn't have done this without you. A huge shout out to Elan, Marc, and Ari for being our personal tech support! You guys rule. And to all of our friends and colleagues who supported us along the way, thank you for believing in us and this workbook.

We would like to voice our tremendous gratitude for all of our friends who read and reviewed our workbook. Our workbook is 100% better because of your feedback and edits. Dr. Sarah Simmons, you are a unicorn of a reviewer. Your insights took our workbook to the next level, and you have our undying love and appreciation! We are so grateful to Dr. Wendy Davis for your time and insightful input on the book, thank you for your wisdom. Sara Krelstein and Marlo Surovsky, thank you for your detailed and thorough edits, they were exactly what we needed at the perfect time. Peggy Nosti, thank you for being such an ally. We appreciate your experience and for being the founder of the Blue Project; your feedback on our workbook was invaluable. Pec Indman, thank you for your ongoing cheerleading, support, and encouragement throughout our writing process! We are grateful to you as well for your book Beyond the Blues with Dr. Shoshana Bennett. Thank you also to Dr. Alison Reminick, Dr. Maria Elswick, Dr. Jay Goldberg, Dr. Kirstin Lee, and Dr. Kat (Katayune Kaeni) for providing support for our project. Thank you also to Gretchen Mallios for your support for this workbook from the beginning. Thank you to Dr. Rebecca Moore for your help with resources in the UK, you are an invaluable wealth of information. And thanks to Joyce Wanderi and Samoina Wangui in Kenya for your help with local resources. Dr. Christine Padesky and Dr. Alyssa Sepinwall, we are beyond grateful for your support and advice on becoming published, your practical tips were so needed. Amy Creager Katz and Ellen Creager, thank you for your tangible support and help! Amy Thompson Kneuppel, Jessica Brody, and Rebecca Barr, your feedback on Chapter 14 was invaluable and we honor your real-life experiences that helped us improve that chapter. Heather Capell Bramble, Dr. Joy Francisco, Dr. Stacy Bonds, Gail Jackson, Nazrie Ray, and Helene Creager Ray, thank you for your brilliant feedback on Chapter 11. Your input was so helpful and we are grateful for your perspectives and lived experiences. And a huge thank you to Heather Evans, Ellie Duncan, Upasruti Biswas, Monica Matthews, Lauren Ellis, and our team at Routledge. We are appreciative we were paired with such patient and positive people throughout this process. You are great teammates.

We would also be remiss if we did not acknowledge all the published authors and therapists in this field who have inspired us, taught us, and laid the pathway for us to write this workbook. Authors like Karen Kleiman, Pec Indman, Dr. Pamela Wiegartz, and Dr. Shoshana Bennett are Wonder Women and have inspired us in our careers. We thank you! And lastly, this book would not be possible without all of the parents who have experienced Perinatal Mood and Anxiety Disorders and emotional changes when having a baby. We know this is so hard, and we think you're amazing.

Epigraph Acknowledgments
Chapter 1: Used by permission of Nikita Gill
Chapter 6: Copyright © Anne Lamott, used by permission of The Wylie Agency LLC
Chapter 9: Copyright © Fred Rogers, used by permission of The Fred Rogers Company
Chapter 11: Used by permission of Zawadi Nyong'o
Chapter 12: Used by permission of Kristin Neff
Chapter 13: Used by permission of Alexandra Elle
Chapter 15: Used by permission of Habeeb Akande
Chapter 16: Prince Caspian by CS Lewis © copyright CS Lewis Pte Ltd 1951. Used with permission.

**Part I**

# Helpful Information – Empowering You with Education

# CHAPTER 1

# HOW TO GET THE MOST OUT OF THIS WORKBOOK

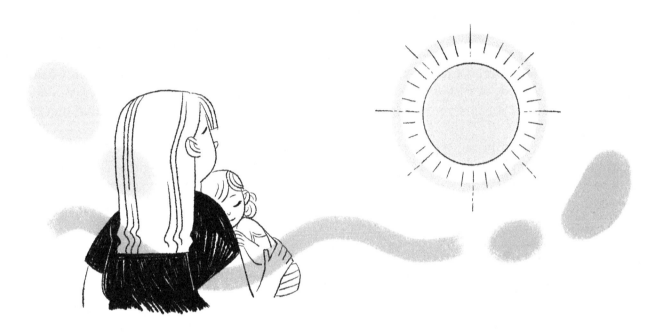

The world has gone dark more times than you or your mother or your grandmother can remember. And every hurricane that was meant to be the end of it all has instead ended in sunshine again. So, believe me when I say: You will survive this. And the next one too.

*- World's End*, by Nikita Gill

DOI: 10.4324/9781003144021-2

Welcome to our book, and we are so glad that you found it! Whether you are pregnant or a postpartum parent, a mental health clinician, an advocate or someone worried about a loved one going through this potentially tough time, we are glad you are here. You are not alone.

Let's face it. It is really normal to feel like your moods are all over the place during your pregnancy and after having a baby. It can be common to be frustrated with the emotions you are experiencing, and maybe you are even a bit freaked out. You might wonder if you will ever be your normal self again (or even wonder if you are experiencing something more serious, like Postpartum or Postnatal Depression that you keep hearing about).

In our practices, pregnant and postpartum women often ask us: "Why am I feeling this way?" "What did I do to cause this?" and "What is wrong with me?" Women often prepare so much for their pregnancies. Some dream about them since childhood, fantasizing about how they will feel, act, and look, and certainly no one dreams about the depression and anxiety they may experience.

Have you found that your partner's chewing is driving you nuts all of a sudden? Do you find yourself crying at absolutely nothing or cheesy commercials? Or more seriously, have you struggled to get out of bed or found worries going round and around in your head like a hamster wheel? What we're getting at is that **all women experience some change in their moods during pregnancy and after having a baby.** With this workbook, we will help you manage whatever emotions you are experiencing. We will also give you strategies to address symptoms that have a more significant impact on your functioning.

Whatever you are experiencing is **common and treatable**. You are not alone. Mood changes are typical and approximately 15–21% of women experience depression and anxiety symptoms during and after pregnancy (Wisner et al., 2013) and wait for it … even 10% of new dads and partners experience these symptoms too (Paulson & Bazemore, 2010; Trenton et al., 2005).

## Did You Know?

- The label "Postpartum Depression" is misleading.

- Mood symptoms can actually occur during pregnancy, not just in the postpartum period.

- Anxiety symptoms are actually more common than depression symptoms both during and after pregnancy.

- Currently, the descriptor is "Perinatal Mood and Anxiety Disorders."

Sadly, many women do not receive help for these symptoms (Barney et al., 2006; Byrne, 2000; Corrigan, 2004). These symptoms can last well over a year if untreated and there is no reason for women to suffer alone or for a prolonged period of time (Thurgood et al., 2009). These emotions you might be experiencing can be painful. But most of the time these are **temporary and treatable,** and we celebrate your first steps toward taking care of yourself! Through this workbook, you will see you are not alone, and you deserve to feel better. This workbook will help you get there.

You may have mild mood changes that come and go (and do not greatly impact your functioning) or more severe symptoms that have really thrown you for a loop and meet the criteria for an actual Perinatal Mood and Anxiety Disorder (PMAD). We will go into the difference between them in the next chapter. For now, we want to introduce you to our workbook so that you can get the most out of it and learn skills to navigate through what can be a difficult time.

## WHY This Book

We both specialize in perinatal mental health and much of our practices are made up of pregnant and postpartum parents. We found that there are so many great books for pregnant and post-partum women out there, but our clients were often sheepishly (or adamantly) admitting to us that they were having a hard time reading some of them because they lacked the concentration needed to conquer a weighty book; sleep deprivation does a number on attention span! It's quite difficult to slog through even the best book when you're so frazzled you barely remember the last time you went to the bathroom or are so tired you keep nodding off when you're up feeding the baby.

We started working together on creating and sharing the exercises we often use with clients, and our "labor of love" began. We wanted to create a workbook with small, readable sections that you could pick up and put down and that interweaves easily with your busy life (and exhausted brain!). We wanted you to have concrete strategies in order to make small changes in your mood over time. Over many, many cups of coffee, technical growing pains with document sharing sites and good old fashioned writing marathon sessions, this workbook was created.

Mostly, we want you to know that it is ok to not feel ok during this time. It is common to not feel ok. You are not alone and by working on yourself you will get better.

## HOW to Use This Book

We get it. You are probably either pregnant "out to here", sleep deprived with a new baby, or just trying to manage being a new parent. It is common for pregnant and new parents to get overwhelmed. In addition, you may be noticing a tremendous shift in your mood and wondering if you will ever get YOU back. This workbook was designed to be used "as needed" – you do not need to read it from cover to cover (though don't let us stop you!). This is not a one-size-fits-all workbook. It is designed to help you with what *you* are going through.

Work on activities at your own pace because we know you're exhausted and might have a very small concentration span at this point. We get it. We designed the workbook activities with this "squirrel brain" in mind.

This workbook can be used alone. It is designed to be user friendly so that you can work on the activities by yourself. However, we recommend that if you identify as having symptoms of a PMAD, that you work with a therapist, in which case this workbook can be a helpful adjunct to therapy and/or medication. How can you identify if you're having symptoms of a PMAD? Please go to Chapter 4: Risk Factors and Screening. Where can you find professional help? Please go to the Resources Chapter.

And, of course, if you are having any serious thoughts requiring immediate help, which include urges to harm yourself or somebody else, then this workbook is not for you right now. Even though these thoughts can be frightening, they are treatable. If you are experiencing these thoughts or urges, please call your doctor, your local emergency number, or one of the following numbers:

**US National Suicide Hotline 1-800-273-8255**

**UK Samaritans Crisis Line 116 123**

**Text HOME to 741741 to connect with a crisis counselor in the US and Canada, 85258 in the UK, and 50808 in Ireland.**

## How Would I Know If I Need Immediate Help?

- If you are having any urges to hurt yourself or anyone else.

- If you are hearing or seeing things that other people are not.

- If you are not able to consistently sleep or eat.

- If you are not able to take care of your own or your baby's basic needs.

## A Note on Examples

We use a lot of examples throughout the book so that you can feel validated and know that you are not alone. We sometimes use our friends' stories with permission, though purposefully chose not to use our clients' stories in order to protect their privacy. However, after forty plus years of practice between us, there may accidentally be some unintentional similarities with prior clients' lives. We are grateful to all of our clients; you inspire us and working with you has been a gift.

## A Note on Language

We purposefully wrote an inclusive workbook that any new parent can use after having a baby, or upon becoming a new parent. We also recognize that there are many types of parents and numerous paths toward becoming a parent. We want all parents to feel represented in this book. Because the majority of research on perinatal mental health is focused on cisgender mothers, as a result, we often use the term "moms and mothers" throughout this book. However, we do try to use the terms "parents and partners" as much as possible and try to use the most updated language at the time of writing this book. We do recognize that there is a significant need for more research on the impact of perinatal mental health on ALL parents, particularly with the intersectionality of mental health on marginalized and underserved communities. For example, there is a lack of thorough research on perinatal mental health with transgender parents. We are hopeful that as inclusivity is more standard, the research will reflect this as well.

However you became a parent and however you found our workbook, we are thrilled you are here, and we imagine you are eager to get some help. In the next chapter we will provide you with information about mood changes in pregnancy and the postpartum period, including perinatal mood and anxiety disorders, so you can better understand what you may be struggling with and learn some constructive ways to deal with it. This workbook can help you get back to being you!

# CHAPTER 2

# WHAT'S GOING ON WITH ME?

## *BREAKING DOWN THE DIFFERENCE BETWEEN BABY BLUES AND PERINATAL MOOD AND ANXIETY DISORDERS*

Bethany Warren, LCSW, PMH-C
Beth Creager Berger, Ph.D.

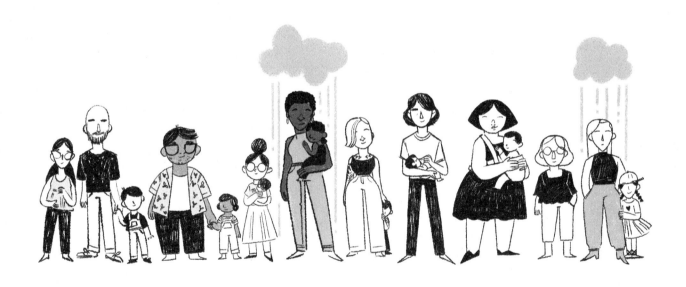

I wish I could show you when you are lonely or in darkness, the astonishing light of your own being.

- *My Brilliant Image*, by Hafiz of Shiraz

DOI: 10.4324/9781003144021-3

Real talk here: how many of you were expecting that during your maternity leave you would be cranking out some adorable birth announcements and going to the park every day while wearing that cute baby-wearing contraption that you got at your baby shower? How many of you thought you could meet your girlfriends for coffee, start a Mommy and Me Yoga class, and rock those adorable stretchy pants you've been dying to get back into after baby?

And how many of you expected to be knocked down by tremendous fears, intrusive thoughts about horrible stuff happening to your baby, or a deep depression that just won't lift?

You did not expect ANY of this. THIS is not what you signed up for, and it is not your fault.

You may think that what you are going through is completely abnormal, but did you know it is really common? It's ok if you didn't. Nobody posts about their miserable experiences on social media, showing themselves in the same pj's for three days, after they've just cried in the shower then yelled at their kids. Instead, they slap a pretty filter on their best selves and project THAT to the world. And so everybody feels alone. When we compare our insides to other people's outsides, we torture ourselves.

---

### Did You Know?

- PMADs are the most common complication of pregnancy with around one out of five women developing a Perinatal Mood and Anxiety Disorder.

- The second and third most common complications of pregnancy are gestational diabetes (cdc. gov) and pregnancy induced hypertension, both of which affects roughly one out of ten to twenty women (Hutcheon, Lisonkova, & Joseph, 2011).

---

Learning about what you are going through can help you feel better and provide validation. We have to talk about it! Early detection and treatment of your changing moods are invaluable to aid in a full recovery. Education can help new parents prepare for what to expect, because, as you now know (but perhaps did not expect), having a baby is not always a joyful experience.

In fact, at times, it can feel defeating and anxiety producing, and super depressing. So early education can aid you to anticipate the support you may need before and after the baby is born.

However, if you are reading this workbook you may find you were not as prepared or knowledgeable for your changing mood as you would have liked. That is OK! You are educating yourself now. Just knowing about the changes in mood that can happen during this time can help you recognize symptoms and allow you to get the help you need.

---

### Did You Know?

- Even adoptive mothers can experience mood changes after becoming a parent!

- Research shows that during the first year after bringing baby home, adoptive mothers showed similar rates of depression symptoms as postpartum women (Mott, Schiller, Richards, O'Hara, & Stuart, 2011).

---

## Baby Blues

Contrary to some social media posts, for most new mothers, the first few weeks after having a baby are a time of mixed emotion. Approximately 80% of new mothers experience what is called the "baby blues" within the first few days of having their baby (Henshaw, 2003). Whether it is the first or the ninth time you have had a baby, postpartum hormonal adjustments are a normal part of the postpartum recovery experience. It is important to note that it is common to experience mood swings following the birth of a child and these symptoms can last up to around two to three weeks postpartum. Baby Blues symptoms can include:

- tearfulness and/or crying for seemingly no reason

- sadness

- anxiety

- irritability

- restlessness

- difficulty sleeping (even when the baby is sleeping)

- poor concentration

- loss or increase of appetite

*Lorena delivered her daughter by epidural-assisted vaginal delivery after many hours of active labor and pushing. She was exhausted and grateful for the nurses' help in the hospital with teaching her how to breastfeed, helping her with her perineum care and even basic recovery and hygiene. She didn't remember ever being so tired! The next several days seemed to pass by in a blur of feedings, bursts of naps and visitors, and before she knew it, she was home. She felt so different, and could burst into tears at the littlest thing, and she often found herself both crying and feeling intense joy with her new baby at the same time. Lorena felt impatient with her partner who was trying her best to help her but of course couldn't rescue her from the land of sore nipples and exhaustion as her partner was also so tired and overwhelmed. As the next few weeks went on though, Lorena started to feel like she was getting into a new groove: she was crying less, able to sleep more, and though she was still so tired, she no longer felt like she was such a zombie.*

## What Causes the Baby Blues?

You know how once you had a baby, you seemed to cry at anything even though you weren't necessarily sad? Or, how you might have been fine one moment, and then were suddenly super anxious about taking a shower and leaving the baby alone for three minutes? The sudden hormonal changes that occur post-delivery significantly influence the mood swings you are experiencing. This period of time is often called the Baby Blues. You are also going through the biggest change in your life! Your world has just blown up and these major life changes are also understandably going to affect your mood as well.

### Did You Know?

- Immediately after childbirth, your hormone levels drop rapidly (Yim et al., 2015).

- These changes can trigger temporary feelings of sadness and anxiety and even longer lasting mood changes.

- Although you can experience hormonal changes up to one year post delivery, the moods associated with the "Baby Blues" usually lessen within the first two weeks after the baby is born.

## So How Will I Know If Something Is More Serious With Me?

Let's help you figure this out. This workbook can be tailored specifically for you. We will go over some more information here and in Chapter 3, and then in Chapter 4, you will have a chance to take some screening questionnaires to further assess your mood symptoms.

Some women continue to experience mood changes longer than a few weeks after delivery (or even start to feel "off" several months after having a baby. We'll talk about this delayed onset of symptoms later). Perinatal Mood and Anxiety Disorders (what we'll refer to as "PMADs" from here on out) is an umbrella term to describe several ways that a person can feel during and after pregnancy. We will go over the diagnoses briefly here, more thoroughly in Chapter 3, and when you take your screening questionnaires in Chapter 4, you can see how impactful your symptoms are.

At the end of this chapter, you will also have a place to review your current symptoms. Chapters 2 and 3 help to clarify what may have been confusing about what you have been feeling. By having a better idea of what you are dealing with, you can develop a plan about how to manage these symptoms.

## So What Are Perinatal Mood and Anxiety Disorders?

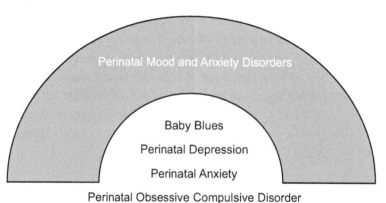

Perinatal Mood and Anxiety Disorders

Baby Blues

Perinatal Depression

Perinatal Anxiety

Perinatal Obsessive Compulsive Disorder

Perinatal Posttraumatic Stress Disorder

Perinatal Bipolar Disorder

Perinatal Psychosis

Approximately one in five new mothers experiences a PMAD, yet, up to 50% of new mothers will not seek treatment (O'Hara & Wisner, 2014; CDC, 2008). We commend you for seeking help through this book! One in ten new dads experience PMADs as well (Paulson & Bazemore, 2010), and while there are still not many statistics at the time of the writing of this book for rates of PMADs in same-sex partners, there is some research highlighting perinatal mood disorders in same-sex parents (Maccio & Pangburn, 2011). Some research does show that lesbian mothers have a higher incidence of PMADs than heterosexual mothers (Ross, Steele, Goldfinger, & Strike, 2007). Clearly more research in this area is necessary.

We also know that there is a significant disparity of PMADs in parents of color, with more Black and Latina women likely to have Perinatal Mood and Anxiety symptoms but less likely to be screened than their White counterparts (Kozhimannil et al., 2011). We explore the impacts of culture and identity further in Chapter 11, and in 12, we talk even more about the impact of perinatal mood symptoms on partners.

> ### Did You Know?
>
> - The most common times of onset of Perinatal Mood and Anxiety Disorders are during pregnancy, immediately after birth, or typically within the first six months after delivery (Gaynes et al., 2005).
>
> - There can be a delayed onset, however, typically starting around the time of other hormonal adjustments such as starting hormonal birth control, the first menstrual period after baby, and when weaning from breastfeeding.

Without treatment, the symptoms from these disorders can last beyond a year and can be quite distressing. However, most PMADs are treatable (Woolhouse et al., 2015; O'Hara et al., 2000), and there are many coping skills that can be learned to help reduce the symptoms of these disorders.

The label "postpartum or postnatal depression" is a misnomer. *Perinatal* is a more inclusive term, which means both during the pregnancy and postpartum period. We now also use the term *Mood and Anxiety Disorders* to include all of the disorders that a woman may experience during this time. For example, a new mom may be experiencing debilitating symptoms of anxiety. She may exhibit worry over not being a good enough mom. This is a common and normal thought among new moms. You may even have heard celebrities such as Serena Williams and Brooke Shields bravely discussing thoughts like this that they experienced. While anxiety and depression are the most commonly discussed mood changes parents experience around this time, there are also several other mood symptoms that parents can encounter, and we will go into those in the next chapter in more depth.

## So, What's the Difference Between Baby Blues and a PMAD?

As we mentioned above, it is incredibly common for most new mothers to experience hormonal fluctuations after having a baby which often manifests as mood changes, tearfulness, etc., within the first few weeks after delivery. It can be common for you to cry at the drop of a hat after the birth of your baby and to be fearful that you are experiencing depression.

However, the biggest difference between the transitional hormonal period we call the "Baby Blues" and a perinatal mood or anxiety disorder is a matter of ***duration, intensity, and frequency*** . By that we mean, EVERY parent is anxious at times. But if she is so anxious that her racing thoughts have lasted months (*duration)*, are so intense she often cannot focus on anything else and interrupts her sleep (*intensity),* and has these racing thoughts throughout the day *(frequency),* this may be more than due to a hormonal adjustment.

**Duration***:* Any symptoms lasting roughly longer than 2 weeks, or symptoms that are not changing or improving.

**Example:** *Zoe is so sad and it doesn't seem to be lifting. She looks back over the last month and can't remember many happy days, in fact, every day seems to feel so heavy.*

**Intensity:** Any symptoms that are so intense they are interfering with your functioning (see below for more information on what this might look like).

**Example:** *Zoe's sadness is so heavy at this point that she now isolates from others and has no motivation to participate in things that used to bring her joy. She has been skipping the drop off line at her son's school in case she happens to run into anyone she knows. She's worried about having to make up an excuse for ditching out on her friends but she just can't muster the energy to hang out with anyone anymore.*

**Frequency:** Any symptoms that happen so frequently they are noteworthy, or distracting you throughout the day.

**Example:** *Zoe has been crying so much! She would never have thought of herself as a crier and now it seems like she could just cry so easily. Plus, she is so irritable and seems to explode at the littlest thing. Her husband is going to need a support group himself; he feels like he has to constantly walk on eggshells around her.*

Regardless of what you are experiencing, this can be a difficult time and we are glad you've picked up this workbook. You can find relief by building skills to manage whatever it is you are feeling.

## How Will I Know If My Symptoms Are Interfering With My Functioning?

You may feel like you are functioning pretty well overall but just don't feel like yourself: the baby is taken care of, you are showering, eating, etc., but you just don't feel well. You may feel down, anxious, or are struggling with obsessive thoughts, for example. You don't have to have a full-blown psychiatric diagnosis in order to suffer, right?

However, your symptoms MAY be impacting your functioning. New moms, no matter how many months after having a baby, may find that their mood changes interfere with their functioning or impact their ability to take care of their baby or other children. Additionally, we find that many moms with mood changes during this time struggle with taking care of some of their own needs. Some parents may actually have a psychiatric diagnosis and we will review some of the common PMADs in the next chapter. The *Diagnostic Statistical Manual of Mental Disorders*, fifth edition (DSM-5) is a guide therapists use to help form a psychiatric diagnosis (American Psychiatric Association, 2013). Unfortunately, the DSM is quite narrow in its definition of PMADS. However, our workbook is not merely meant for the new parent who meets full criteria for a psychiatric diagnosis. It is meant for ANY new parent who is struggling at all. This workbook is for you. Whatever you are experiencing, we will help you develop some skills to improve your functioning and help you feel better. In the meantime, it's important to identify HOW you are being impacted and in what areas you are struggling.

## Some Signs Your Mood Symptoms May Be Interfering With Your Functioning (Check Any That Apply to You):

☐ You are neglecting your own needs (i.e. not showering or not eating regularly)

☐ You aren't able to sleep when your baby is sleeping (you can't shut your thoughts down)

☐ You have stopped doing activities that used to bring you happiness (not because you're a busy parent but because you simply don't feel like it)

☐ You are isolating from others

☐ You are having a difficult time completing tasks or unable to focus.

☐ You are losing your temper easily, or your anger is distracting or is impacting your relationships

☐ You don't have the energy to change or feed your baby, or are so anxious about doing so that you avoid many childrearing activities

## So, How ARE You Doing?

What ARE you feeling? Take a minute and check the feelings you've experienced over the past two weeks that have been impacting you.

**Please Put a Check by Any Symptoms or Issues You Are Currently Experiencing, or Have Experienced Regularly Over the Past Two Weeks**.

Racing thoughts _____ Worrying/anxiety _____ Panic attacks_____ Fears _____

Difficulty concentrating _____ Change in appetite _____ Loss of interest in activities _____

Irritability _____ Anger_____ Depression _____ Sadness _____ Hopelessness _____

Sleep problems _____ Loss of energy_____ Weight changes _____ Memory changes _____

Grief/loss _____ Tearfulness _____ Lack of motivation _____ Low self-esteem _____

Easily frustrated _____ Hyperactivity _____ Euphoria _____ Impulsivity _____

Relationship issues _____ Sexual issues _____ Mood swings _____ Feeling empty _____

Flashbacks _____ Nightmares _____ Disorientation _____ Confusion _____

*Seeing things others do not _____ *Self-harm _____ *Suicidal thoughts _____

*Hearing things others do not _____ *Feeling paranoid _____

*If you have checked any of the last two rows of symptoms, it is important for you to seek outside help with a professional right now because you need the additional support. The Resources chapter has some good recommendations.*

**What Was This Experience Like in Marking Down the Symptoms You Are Feeling?**

_____
_____
_____

**Were Any of Your Symptoms Above Surprising to You?**

_____
_____
_____

It can be really useful to identify what you are feeling in order to create a plan for your recovery.

**When Did Your Symptoms Start? What Does Delayed Onset Mean?**

It is most common to experience mood changes during pregnancy and after having a baby. However, some women will also experience a delayed onset of their symptoms. As mentioned at the beginning of this chapter, it can be very common for mood symptoms to start at several different times **(check when you noticed yours starting or worsening)**:

☐   During pregnancy

☐   After giving birth

☐   When starting hormonal birth control again

☐   When you got your first period after having your baby

☐   When you weaned breastfeeding

As you may notice, these are all times of hormonal disruption and change. Many women may not have known that these are common times for changing moods as well, so are surprised when they are feeling "off" during their pregnancy or many months after having a baby. Imagine if you stop breastfeeding when your baby is 14 months old, and that's when you start feeling depressed or anxious! It can be hard to link this back to perinatal mood changes if you did not know that a delayed onset of symptoms can happen. These feelings can be further worsened if you are stressed about going back to work or making difficult decisions around childcare. It can be empowering to be educated about why you are feeling the way you are feeling.

Now that you have learned more about the difference between the "Baby Blues" and other mood symptoms falling under Perinatal Mood and Anxiety Disorders, let's review the rest of the PMADs. In the next chapter, we will go into the other Perinatal Mood and Anxiety Disorder symptoms in more depth so you can learn more about what you're experiencing and start forming strategies to help yourself feel better.

## Important Takeaway

•   Perinatal Mood and Anxiety Disorders are the most common complication of pregnancy, with one in five mothers experiencing these mood changes.

•   One in ten fathers and same-sex partners can experience these mood changes as well.

•   You can help figure out the severity of your mood symptoms by checking in with yourself about the duration, intensity, and frequency of your symptoms.

•   Your symptoms might have started during pregnancy or even had a delayed onset months after having a baby.

•   Regardless of what you are experiencing, this workbook can help you!

# CHAPTER 3

## LEARNING MORE ABOUT YOUR MOODS

### *NO, SERIOUSLY, WHAT'S GOING ON WITH ME?*

Bethany Warren, LCSW, PMH-C
Beth Creager Berger, Ph.D.

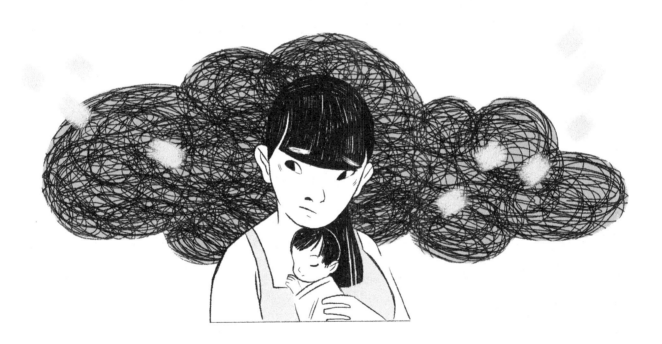

Even the darkest night will end and the sun will rise

- *Les Misérables*, by Victor Hugo

DOI: 10.4324/9781003144021-4

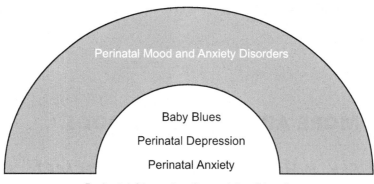

Perinatal Mood and Anxiety Disorders

Baby Blues

Perinatal Depression

Perinatal Anxiety

Perinatal Obsessive Compulsive Disorder

Perinatal Posttraumatic Stress Disorder

Perinatal Bipolar Disorder

Perinatal Psychosis

Let's face it, what you're experiencing sucks. Luckily you aren't going to be experiencing ALL of these mood symptoms that we talk about below, but we wanted to have one place where we could lay it all out for you to read in case you're interested in doing a deep dive. Information is power, right? Some people like to learn a lot about what they're going through and find it helps them feel better while some people just want to be told what to do about it. Wherever you land is fine. This chapter is going to go over all the Perinatal Mood and Anxiety Disorder symptoms and give examples, so if you want to learn more, stick around! At the end of the chapter, we have some brief activities for you to be able to start to identify what emotions, feelings, and thoughts you are having. This is a helpful way to start creating a plan towards feeling better. If you'd like to join us in Chapter 4 to further assess your own symptoms, we'll see you there.

## Perinatal Depression

Are you feeling super sad, irritable, or sluggish? Do you ever feel like you're swimming in molasses or your brain is super foggy? You are not alone. One out of seven women feel the same way. Perinatal Depression symptoms can start during pregnancy, after birth, and there also can be a delayed onset as well of up to around two years after giving birth (Gaynes et al., 2005). Depression symptoms can present alone or in combination with anxiety (we like to think of them like thunder and lighting, they often show up together).

### Common Symptoms of Perinatal Depression Can Also Include:

- Depressed mood most of the day (sad, hopeless, tearful)

- Feelings of anger, irritability, or rage

- Markedly diminished interest in pleasurable activities

- A decrease or increase in appetite nearly every day or a significant weight loss or gain

- Not being able to sleep or sleeping more than normal (Note: not being able to sleep when the baby is sleeping is a red flag that something may be going on with you; not sleeping because you can't shut your brain off is different than not being able to sleep because you're up with the baby).

- Fatigue or loss of energy (not due to a lack of sleep)

- Diminished ability to think or concentrate

- Feelings of worthlessness or guilt

- Recurrent thoughts of death or recurrent suicidal thoughts either with or without a specific plan*

- Urges to harm your baby* **

*If you are experiencing suicidal thoughts or urges to harm yourself or anyone else, you need to seek professional help right away. Emergency resources are listed in the Resources Chapter at the end of the book. While not every parent who experiences depression will have suicidal thoughts, we want you to know this is treatable and you are not alone.
** Although this is rare, it is important for us to acknowledge it.

*Jasmin was just so irritable. Ever since she had her son, she wanted to rip somebody's head off; she felt like she could fully understand that term "mama bear". She loved him very much but really felt like she hated everybody else. She couldn't help but compare herself to other moms, and felt like other mothers in the stores and at the park had it all together. Why was she struggling so much with breastfeeding, getting out of the house, and enjoying motherhood? Don't get her wrong, she LOVED her son, but it made her so angry when she saw how perfect everyone else was. She cried sometimes when she was by herself, but it was so hard to reach out to others because surely nobody else would feel the same. Plus, the brain fog! Jasmin found it so hard to do even the simplest of tasks. Getting a load of laundry done was laughable, she would get so easily distracted, was exhausted, and she had no motivation to do it anyway. And forget about doing anything that used to make her happy. Nothing seemed to work anymore. She couldn't help but wonder, is this what motherhood looks like, or is it just her?*

# Perinatal Anxiety

Have you ever been carrying your baby down the stairs and had a fearful thought about dropping her? Almost everyone does. However, if that thought doesn't leave and keeps rolling around like on a hamster wheel, you might be experiencing a form of anxiety. Perinatal Anxiety is super common and can affect more than 15% of pregnant and postpartum women (Fairbrother et al., 2016) and often includes either physical symptoms (i.e. panic attacks, restlessness, jitteriness, or feelings of excess energy) and/ or worrying (i.e. racing thoughts, feelings of dread, belief that bad things will happen). Behaviorally, this is likely to impact you because the tendency might be to avoid situations that are distressing. For example, if you fear that your baby will have a meltdown when you go to the grocery store, you may want to stay home and isolate. You may dread the worst-case scenarios at all times, picturing horrible things happening, and feeling certain they will. And remember, often times anxiety and depression can go hand in hand, and you may be experiencing symptoms of both simultaneously.

## Perinatal Anxiety Symptoms Can Also Include:

- Constant worry

- Feeling that something bad is going to happen

- Racing thoughts

- Disturbances in sleep (Note: again, not being able to shut your brain down at night is different than being awake with your baby).

- Inability to sit still

- Hypochondriasis (frequent worries about your health or the baby's health)

- Physical symptoms, such as a racing heart, dizziness, shakiness, clamminess, hot flashes, nausea

*Emma just couldn't stop her brain, it was like a hamster wheel going and going nonstop. She was constantly worrying and could always see the worst-case scenario happening. She felt like she was crazy with the things she was afraid of. She stopped telling other people about it because they would look at her funny or say, "don't even think that way", which made her feel awful. "Don't you think I'd stop if I could?" she thought. She felt like an elephant was sitting on her chest. Trying to leave the house with her baby felt impossible. She could easily think of a million things that could go wrong, from the most "benign" like "I will cry and people will judge me" to the most horrific. Looking back, she realized she was always a worrier, but nothing like this. She was able to function before but now Emma felt absolutely paralyzed. And the indecisiveness! It's so hard to even make a simple decision, much less complex ones like when to stop breastfeeding or when to introduce solid foods. She felt so exhausted but it was also impossible to fall asleep; her brain just spun and spun.*

## Perinatal Obsessive-Compulsive Disorder

Do you ever have unwanted, intrusive images of bad things happening to you or your baby? Do you avoid places or situations out of fear that they're either dangerous or distressing (or you don't trust yourself there)? Do you try to control situations by excessive cleaning, obsessive rituals, or counting? Actual Perinatal Obsessive-Compulsive Disorder is not as common as depression or anxiety, 1–3% of mothers have this diagnosis (Russell, Fawcett & Mazmanian, 2007; Zimbaldi et al., 2009). However, it is really common to have some obsessive or intrusive thoughts during the pregnancy and postpartum period even if you don't meet all the criteria for a diagnosis of Perinatal OCD.

### Did You Know?

- Upwards of 40% of moms with anxiety or depression report they also have intrusive and unwanted images that pop into their mind (Zimbaldi et al., 2009).

- More than 90% of ALL mothers report having scary thoughts at some point (Kleiman, 2019)!

Intrusive or obsessive images can often involve imagining harm coming to the baby, yourself or your loved ones. We are choosing not to give specific examples here so that we are not adding more anxiety to your plate. However, suffice it to say, if you have thought about it or pictured it, we have likely heard it from clients, no matter how intense the content. This is not your fault nor would your thoughts rattle us. We will help you learn to manage these thoughts more in Chapter 8.

We all have intrusive images at times. For example, we might have had the experience of driving down the highway next to a truck stacked sky high with objects and we can see in our mind's eye the image of the truck's objects crashing down onto our car. Our heart may start racing a bit, we may even look around to make our exit strategy into another lane if we need, but once we've passed that truck, the image passes as does the distress. With obsessive images and the compulsive avoidance or repetitive checking behavior that sometimes accompanies it, these images do NOT fade, often play on a loop and are quite distressing.

## Symptoms of Perinatal OCD Can Include:

- Obsessions (aka intrusive thoughts or images) are repetitive and persistent thoughts or images related to oneself, the baby or others. These thoughts are unwanted and can be very upsetting.

- Compulsions are actions done in order to reduce the distress related to the obsessions or fears. These actions can be repetitive checking, cleaning, counting, or reordering of things.

- Being horrified or scared about the intrusive thoughts or images

- Avoidance of any disturbing or distressing situation that occurs in the obsessive thoughts

- Fear of being left alone with the infant

- Hypervigilance in protecting the infant

- Parents with Perinatal OCD know that their thoughts are bizarre and are unlikely to ever act on them. In fact, they will often say that they never want any harm to come to their baby and would never purposefully hurt their baby, which is why the thoughts are so disturbing to them.

*Kim felt like she was going crazy. The images that would flash in her mind about horrific things happening to her baby boy were like something out of a horror movie, and certainly a movie she would never want to watch. She would be doing something completely normal like cooking dinner and then WHAM! A horrible image would pop in her mind and she would see it play it out – the images were so vivid it felt so real like it could actually happen. When the images involved situations she could prevent like using the stairs or knives in her kitchen, she would do everything she could to avoid those objects. She worried she might lose control and do the things that she saw in those horrible "movies" in her mind. She felt such shame about these awful images that she was fearful to tell anyone. Even though she loved her son desperately and would NEVER want to harm him, in fact would do anything to protect him (including avoiding the ever-growing list of objects!), she was so scared if she told anyone, they would think she was crazy and take her son away from her.*

## Perinatal Posttraumatic Stress Disorder (PPTSD)

Did you experience a traumatic or distressing birth experience? Was your pregnancy difficult or did you have postpartum complications? Did you find breastfeeding so challenging that nursing became really triggering and anxiety producing?

Perinatal Posttraumatic Stress Disorder is often caused by a traumatic experience during fertility treatments, pregnancy complications, delivery, after delivery of the infant, or even during the postpartum period such as distress with breastfeeding. Anywhere between 9% and 41% of women can experience symptoms of Perinatal Posttraumatic Stress Disorder following childbirth and 34% of women report having a traumatic birth experience (Beck, 2013; Anderson, 2010).

### Symptoms of Perinatal Posttraumatic Stress Disorder Can Include:

- Intrusive re-experiencing of a past traumatic event (replaying it in your mind over and over)

- Flashbacks or nightmares in which you feel like the event is still happening

- Desire to avoid anything associated with the event, including thoughts, feelings, people, places, and details of the event (like wanting to avoid the doctor's office or hospital)

- Persistent increased arousal (irritability, difficulty sleeping, hypervigilance, exaggerated startle response)

- Anxiety or panic attacks

- Feeling of a sense of unreality and detachment (either "I'm not real" or "my world doesn't feel real")

- Triggers of situations, sounds, feelings or emotions reminding you of your experience (i.e. the hospital itself, noises similar to your IV machine, a person who looks like a hospital staff member involved in the delivery, etc.)

We find that women who experience trauma around the reproductive period may or may not be able to identify it as actual trauma. Trauma is subjective. This means that an experience can be traumatic regardless of the outcome. Do you know anyone that had a difficult delivery experience and yet feels fairly positive about her birth overall? How about the opposite: do you know a mom (or perhaps you yourself) who had a difficult birth experience, and despite a good outcome with the baby, she feels like a failure, or she even still feels unsafe and scared?

PTSD (Posttraumatic Stress Disorder) symptoms can be triggered by a frightening event in which there is perceived or real danger. This means that you may have a beautiful happy baby, or you yourself may have escaped great harm but may still feel traumatized. You do not have to have full PTSD symptoms to have experienced trauma during this time and for your experience to have a negative impact on you. Some common reproductive traumas can be **(check any that may pertain to you):**

☐  Having had an emergency cesarean section

☐  Your baby was in distress and/or you were separated from your baby

☐  You delivered your baby delivery prematurely and/or your baby spent time in the Neonatal Intensive Care Unit

☐  You had an unwanted medicated birth or an unwanted birth experience

☐  You had difficulty with breastfeeding

☐  You experienced high conflict with hospital staff, feeling unsafe or unheard during delivery experience

☐  You may have had a traumatic birth experience itself or perceived your birth experience as being traumatic.

---

### Did You Know?

- Your birth experience can also trigger a past traumatic experience (i.e. a reminder of another traumatic experience from the past).

- This can include incidents such as a prior assault, previous abuse, or even remind you of other times you have felt unsafe or powerless.

- Regardless if you have full PTSD symptoms or some experience of trauma, this is treatable.

---

*Jennifer thought her emergency cesarean section was scary and it felt "unreal" at that time, particularly with all of the people who were crammed into the small space. Everything happened so quickly, and they rushed her daughter out of the Operating Room and to the Neonatal ICU without her even getting to hold her new baby. Yet, it wasn't until she got home that the reality of how bad things could have been really hit her.*

*Everyone in Jennifer's life was telling her to focus on her healthy baby, and they were reminding her to be grateful for how well things turned out. But Jennifer couldn't help but play out the events over and over in her mind. Sometimes she even woke up in a panic, feeling confused about where she was or being so scared about her baby's safety. She didn't even feel reassured once she checked on her daughter in her crib. She noticed the weirdest things, like the ice maker of her fridge now made her jump whereas that sound never bothered her before. She also felt so scared about leaving the house and even the smallest things would "set her off." She would easily become angry at her loved ones trying to help her. Jennifer felt like she was going crazy and if one more person pointed out how lucky she was to have such a good outcome and she should be happy and just move on, she could just scream.*

# Perinatal Bipolar Disorder

Are your moods so unstable and up and down that you don't feel like yourself? Have any of your loved ones told you that they're worried about your extreme mood changes? Do you feel like you just can't "get a grip" on your emotions?

Up to around 20% of women can experience Bipolar symptoms during their pregnancy or after delivering a baby, and this is commonly misdiagnosed as only depression (Wisner et al., 2013). In fact, 56% of women previously diagnosed with "Postpartum depression" actually had Bipolar Disorder, so it's important to be educated about the symptoms. (Sharma & Khan, 2010). People with Bipolar Disorder experience at least one episode of mania (which is an elevated or euphoric mood which can include grandiosity, a decreased need for sleep, and racing thoughts for at least a week) or hypomania (for at least four days), and at least one episode of depression (American Psychiatric Association, 2013).

## Symptoms of Perinatal Bipolar Disorder Can Include:

- Mood changes from highs to lows

- Depression

- Euphoria or feeling high energy

- Irritability or restlessness

- Difficulty sleeping when the baby is sleeping

- Impulsivity

- Psychosis is possible, though less common (such as visual or auditory hallucinations, or seeing or hearing things that are not there)

There are two types of this disorder: Bipolar 1 and Bipolar 2, and both involve depressive moods combined with additional elevated moods. Bipolar 1 Disorder can be more severe with symptoms warranting more immediate assessment and treatment. This can sometimes even include seeing or hearing things that do not exist (these are known as hallucinations). Though less severe, Bipolar 2 Disorder can also include symptoms which need an assessment by a professional. If you suspect any mood changes that feel intolerable, reaching out to a trained provider for a full assessment is always a good idea (see Chapter 4 for further tools to screen your symptoms and the Resources chapter for added help).

*Erica has not felt like herself since starting her third trimester. She noticed she started needing less sleep and initially thought it was what people had prepared her for when they said "your bladder will start waking you up!". But it wasn't like that. It was almost like there was a buzzing inside her. She had energy that was like electricity that wouldn't turn off when she tried to close her eyes. What sleep she got just wasn't good quality sleep. She felt so on edge, too. It was easy to snap at her husband and coworkers and she was easily "road ragey" now. It was like the whole world had become a bunch of idiots.*

*She didn't want to admit it, but she was spending money like crazy too. It didn't seem to be like what her friends called "nesting" and how they were getting ready for their babies; sometimes she would go on big benders and buy a bunch of stuff and it was such a high! But then she would come crashing down afterwards, hiding the receipts from her husband and really spiraling into a self-blame cycle. She would feel so low and that feeling would last days sometimes. Erica tried to talk to her other pregnant friends about this, wondering if this was just pregnancy hormones kicking in at the last minute, but her friends seemed to be feeling such different things, so Erica just stopped asking. She knew what she was feeling was off, but it was hard to put into words.*

# Postpartum Psychosis

Are you feeling as if your world is not real right now, or that even you are not real? Are you hearing or seeing things that others do not? Are you feeling increasingly paranoid? Are you frustrated that others are not sharing in your beliefs or experiencing what you are experiencing?

This can be a very scary and uncertain time. Perhaps this is not even the birth parent that is reading this section, and maybe the partner or loved one of the birth parent has picked up this section to read it. Regardless of who is reading this, we are glad you are here.

If you suspect that you or your loved one are experiencing what is known as Postpartum Psychosis, then please hear us: you have done nothing wrong. This can feel really scary, and it's important you get professional help to feel like yourself again. Working with a perinatal psychiatrist can be a proactive step towards feeling better. Using this workbook alone is not for you right now so please pick it back up after you are working with a qualified professional.

## Symptoms of Postpartum Psychosis Can Include:

- Disorganized or bizarre behavior

- Delusional, paranoid, or irrational bizarre thoughts

- Visual, auditory, or tactile hallucinations (seeing, hearing, or feeling things that are not there)

- Rapidly changing moods

- Loss of appetite

- Thoughts about harming oneself or the baby that are delusional and that the parent does NOT identify as irrational. The difference between psychosis and OCD is that with OCD the parent realizes the thoughts are irrational, they are often quite distressed by the thoughts and images, and they have no intention of harming themselves or the baby. Whereas with psychosis these types of thoughts feel rational to the parent.

Psychosis after having a baby usually has a rapid onset, typically within the first few days or weeks postpartum. This is a rare disorder, affecting 1%–2% of women (VanderKruik et al., 2017), and is a true medical emergency. While this can be a tough thing for you or your loved ones to witness, the positive news about Perinatal Psychosis is that it is responsive to treatment. If you or someone you know is experiencing these symptoms, please help facilitate them getting to professional treatment right away.

## So How Would I Get Help?

Ideas for finding professional help are in the back of the book in our Resources Chapter, or if this feels like a more urgent need, you can go to your closest emergency room and request a psychiatric evaluation.

*Tessa could have sworn she heard the neighbors talking about her at all hours of the night. They were whispering about what a bad mother she was and judging every little thing she was doing. During every diaper she changed, she would hear them narrate the entire operation, critiquing her every move, cruelly commenting on her poor form. She would hear them say what a horrible mom she was, and how she was so unfit to take care of herself, much less a baby. Her partner kept reassuring her that there was no way that the neighbors were able to see through the baby monitor or talk to her but how else could they explain how she could hear them? Plus, when she would go outside, her world felt different, almost like she was in a dream or watching a movie; everything just felt so off.*

## Activity:

We get it. We've just thrown a lot at you. In the next chapter we will give you an opportunity to assess your specific symptoms and figure out how much those symptoms are impacting you on a daily basis.

This will help you determine not only what it is you're needing but also the right plan for you. For now let's look more generally at why you picked up this workbook in the first place. What is bothering you, and what are you currently experiencing? It will be helpful to list some of the things you are feeling and thinking so that you can better understand what you are dealing with.

In our practices, we often find our clients come into their first sessions with so much to share that it can be difficult for some of them to put it into words. It can feel so big and overwhelming that our job can be like a funnel, clarifying and ultimately focusing the session down to the crux of the issue. By writing your core thoughts, feelings, and body sensations, this can better help you identify what you're experiencing right now. In Chapter 7, we'll help you dig deeper into how these thoughts, feelings, and body sensations can all be interconnected.

## EMOTIONS / FEELINGS:

Some of the emotions or feelings I'm having recently are **(circle all that apply within the last month)**:

| | | | | | |
|---|---|---|---|---|---|
| Anger | Frustration | Sadness | Anxiety | Resentment | Overwhelm |
| Grief | Afraid | Disoriented | Jealous | Insecure | Panicked |
| Uncertain | Self-blame | Negative | Desperate | Restless | Self-conscious |
| Happy | Grateful | Proud | Strong | Amazed | Exhilarated |

Other emotions I've been feeling:_____

## PHYSICAL SENSATIONS:

Some of the body or physical sensations I'm experiencing are **(circle all that apply within the last month)**:

| | | | | | |
|---|---|---|---|---|---|
| Low energy | Aching body | Tension | Headaches | Pain | Racing heart |
| Heartburn | Pelvic pain | Nausea | Bleeding | Swelling | Restlessness |

Other body sensations I'm feeling:_____

**NEGATIVE THOUGHTS:** (Examples might be "I'm a bad mom for feeling this way", "Everybody else is doing so much better as a mom than me", "I'm not cut out for this", "What if something bad happens", etc.)

**Some of the negative thoughts I'm currently having are:**

_____
_____
_____
_____
_____
_____
_____
_____
_____
_____

## Important Takeaways

- There are several more Perinatal Mood and Anxiety Disorders (PMADs) than the most commonly known one of Postpartum or Postnatal Depression.

- You might be experiencing symptoms of depression, anxiety, obsessive compulsive disorder, Posttraumatic Stress Disorder, Bipolar Disorder, or psychosis.

- Whatever you are experiencing is temporary and treatable, so it's great you are taking care of yourself and addressing your symptoms!

**CHAPTER 4**

# RISK FACTORS AND SCREENING

## *WHY ME, AND WHAT NEXT?*

**Bethany Warren, LCSW, PMH-C**
**Beth Creager Berger, Ph.D.**

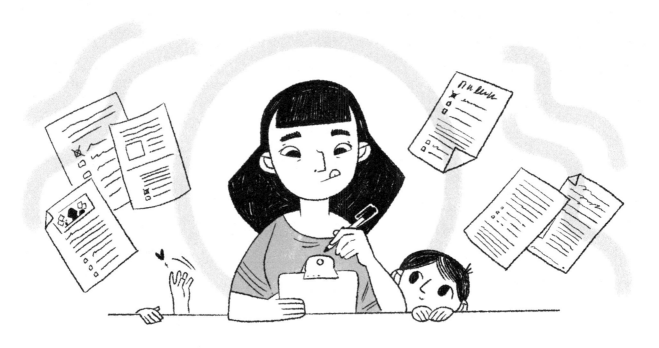

The journey of a thousand miles begins with one step.

- Lao Tzu

DOI: 10.4324/9781003144021-5

We hope that at this point that you might be feeling validated by recognizing some of the symptoms you may be experiencing. You might also be feeling nervous since you are still likely struggling. This is a good time to remind you that **mood changes and mental health disorders around the perinatal period are treatable!** In fact, this is a great time to screen and assess your symptoms further. We have two screening tools below that are the community standard for assessing symptoms of PMADS.

We know this might be intimidating after everything you have just learned, and it may be tempting to either diagnose yourself or avoid thinking about this entirely. However, identifying the baseline of what you are experiencing now can be an important part of your recovery. We also recommend taking these screenings approximately once a month or more to track your progress. If you were to compare yourself to how you were doing yesterday, you may grow discouraged if you did not see much change. But if you compare yourself to where you were a month ago, you will likely see change and growth.

We have two quick tips as you do these: (1) please answer the questions with how you've been feeling within **the last week**, not necessarily today, as symptoms can change so much from day to day; and (2) remember these are for assessing, not diagnosing yourself. The assessments will give you a sense of the extent and severity of your symptoms; however, in order to get a true diagnosis, you need to be evaluated by a mental health professional.

## Edinburgh Postpartum Depression Scale (EPDS):

Even though in the title, this assessment scale says "postpartum", this scale can also be used during pregnancy. As you will see, the questions tend to largely focus on depression-type symptoms and are fairly limited for use with anxiety. The general rule of thumb is that any score above 11 warrants talking to a professional about your symptoms for further assessment. Regardless of your overall score, if you answered anything other than "0" on question #10 (the question about safety), we recommend you talk to a professional immediately as this indicates that what you are experiencing is more serious than anything that should be managed on your own and that you need outside help. You deserve to get the help you need, and you do not need to do this alone. (Again, resources for help are at the back of this book).

**EPDS:**

## EDINBURGH POSTNATAL DEPRESSION SCALE (EDPS)

Please place a CHECK MARK by the answer that comes closest to how you have felt IN THE PAST 7 DAYS – not just how you feel today. Complete all 10 items and find your score by adding each number that you checked. This is a screening test, not a medical diagnosis. If something doesn't feel right, call your health care provider regardless of your score.

| 1. I have been able to laugh and see the funny side of things: | As much as I always could **(0)** | Not quite so much now **(1)** | Definitely not so much now **(2)** | Not at all **(3)** |
|---|---|---|---|---|
| 2. I have looked forward with enjoyment to things: | As much as I ever did **(0)** | Rather less than I used to **(1)** | Definitely less than I used to **(2)** | Hardly at all **(3)** |
| 3. I have blamed myself unnecessarily when things went wrong: | Yes, most of the time **(3)** | Yes, some of the time **(2)** | Not very often **(1)** | No, never **(0)** |
| 4. I have been anxious or worried for no good reason: | No, not at all **(0)** | Hardly ever **(1)** | Yes, sometimes **(2)** | Yes, very often **(3)** |
| 5. I have felt scared or panicky for no good reason: | Yes, quite a lot **(3)** | Yes, sometimes **(2)** | No, not much **(1)** | No, not at all **(0)** |
| 6. Things have been getting to me: | Yes, most of the time I haven't been able to cope at all **(3)** | Yes, sometimes I haven't been coping as well as usual **(2)** | No, most of the time I have coped quite well **(1)** | No, I have been coping as well as ever **(0)** |
| 7. I have been so unhappy that I have had difficulty sleeping: | Yes, most of the time **(3)** | Yes, sometimes **(2)** | No, not very often **(1)** | No, not at all **(0)** |
| 8. I have felt sad or miserable: | Yes, most of the time **(3)** | Yes, quite often **(2)** | Not very often **(1)** | No, not at all **(0)** |
| 9. I have been so unhappy that I have been crying: | Yes, most of the time **(3)** | Yes, quite often **(2)** | Only occasionally **(1)** | No, never **(0)** |
| 10. The thought of harming myself has occurred to me: | Yes, quite often **(3)** | Sometimes **(2)** | Hardly ever **(1)** | Never **(0)** |

Edinburgh Postnatal Depression Scale (EPDS). Adapted from the *British Journal of Psychiatry*, June 1987, vol. 150 by J.L. Cox, J.M. Holden, R. Segovsky.

## Perinatal Anxiety Screening Scale (PASS)

This scale is specifically for anxiety and assesses common fears and worries that parents can experience (intrusive thoughts, general worrying, phobias and fears, etc.). A score of 26 or higher indicates a higher risk of a Perinatal Anxiety Disorder. Again, this is not used for diagnosing a disorder by itself, but a higher score indicates that further assessment can be helpful.

## PASS:

### PERINATAL ANXIETY SCREENING SCALE (PASS)

OVER THE PAST MONTH, how often have you experienced the following? Please tick the response that most closely describes your experience for every question.

| | Not at all (0) | Sometimes (1) | Often (2) | Almost Always (3) |
|---|---|---|---|---|
| 1. Worry about the baby / pregnancy | | | | |
| 2. Fear that harm will come to the baby | | | | |
| 3. A sense of dread that something bad is going to happen | | | | |
| 4. Worry about many things | | | | |
| 5. Worry about the future | | | | |
| 6. Feeling overwhelmed | | | | |
| 7. Really strong fears about things, such as needles, blood, birth, pain, etc. | | | | |
| 8. Sudden rushes of extreme fear or discomfort | | | | |
| 9. Repetitive thoughts that are difficult to stop or control | | | | |
| 10. Difficulty sleeping even when I have the chance to sleep | | | | |
| 11. Having to do things in a certain way or order | | | | |
| 12. Wanting things to be perfect | | | | |
| 13. Needing to be in control of things | | | | |
| 14. Difficulty stopping checking or doing things over and over | | | | |
| 15. Feeling jumpy or easily startled | | | | |
| 16. Concerns about repeated thoughts | | | | |
| 17. Being "on guard" or needing to watch out for things | | | | |
| 18. Upset about repeated memories, dreams or nightmares | | | | |
| 19. Worry that I will embarrass myself in front of others | | | | |
| 20. Fear that others will judge me negatively | | | | |
| 21. Feeling really uneasy in crowds | | | | |
| 22. Avoiding social activities because I might be nervous | | | | |
| 23. Avoiding things which concern me | | | | |
| 24. Feeling detached like you're watching yourself in a movie | | | | |
| 25. Losing track of time and can't remember what happened | | | | |
| 26. Difficulty adjusting to recent changes | | | | |
| 27. Anxiety getting in the way of being able to do things | | | | |
| 28. Racing thoughts making it hard to concentrate | | | | |
| 29. Fear of losing control | | | | |
| 30. Feeling panicky | | | | |
| 31. Feeling agitated | | | | |

The Perinatal Anxiety Screening Scale has been reproduced with the permission of the Authors and the WA Department of Health. Somerville, S., Dedman, K., Hagan, R., Oxnam, E., Wettinger, M., Byrne, S., Coo, S., Doherty, D., Page, A.C. (2014). The Perinatal Anxiety Screening Scale: development and preliminary validation. Archives of Women's Mental Health, DOI: 10.1007/s00737-014-0425-8

## Activity:

Take both the EPDS and the PASS. Now that you've taken the two common screening tools for Perinatal Mood and Anxiety Disorders, please list your scores here:

**EPDS:** _____                    **PASS:** _____

What was that experience like for you? When we have our clients take these screening questionnaires, we like to ask them afterwards if there were any surprises for them, and often, our clients will mention that these questions further confirmed how they've been feeling. In other words, these screening scales often felt validating even if it was a little scary to finally confront what they've been fighting. **What thoughts came up for you as you took the screening questionnaires and saw your scores?** Did you feel any relief? Validation? Shame or self-blame?

_____

_____

_____

_____

*Sandra feels such shame about her feelings of depression. She struggled with infertility for years, plus she had several miscarriages so by the time she adopted her precious baby boy, she finally thought the worst was behind her. But it's not. In fact, even though she loves her son, the world still feels gray and her sadness doesn't seem to lift. She certainly is capable of taking care of him and herself, but she feels like she's moving through molasses, like everything is just harder than it should be. Nothing really brings her joy, and when everyone keeps saying to her "aren't you so happy now?" she feels even more guilt, like she doesn't deserve this moment, or even this baby. It wasn't until her therapist pointed out everything she had been through: all of her losses, her years of infertility treatments, all of her lack of control and struggles, that she was able to piece it all together. It still feels really hard, but at least she's able to find a sliver of compassion with herself: she has been through a huge battle, and she has the scars to prove it. This has been a hard journey.*

You may have already told someone you love what you are going through, or instead, you may be isolated and struggling with this on your own. It can be common for women to tell themselves distorted thoughts, like that they are bad moms, if feeling this way. But this is NOT the case. This is not your fault. You are a good mom, and you are working hard to get better for you and your family. Unfortunately, self-blame, if unchecked, often leads to isolation. However, by even telling ONE safe person what you are experiencing, you can feel unburdened and together you can come up with a plan. Who might you tell? Examples might include a family member who is typically non-judgmental, a friend who has shared difficult things with you before, a girlfriend who also just had a baby, etc.

**One safe person I can identify that I will tell about what I'm going through is:**

_____

**Risk Factors:**
Now let's talk about WHY this is happening. In our practices, pregnant and post-partum parents often ask us: "Why am I feeling this way?" "What did I do to cause this?" and "What is wrong with me?" Women often prepare so much for their pregnancies. Some dream about them since childhood, fantasizing about

how they will feel, act, and look. Certainly no one dreams about the depression and anxiety they may experience. Having mood changes during or after pregnancy can be devastating. Often, self-blame can be a common reaction if a woman does not have information about why this happened. The answer is unfortunately complicated, and we know that perinatal mood changes are a complex "perfect storm" of biological, psychological, and environmental factors. In Chapter 10 we will talk about all the amazing changes your brain is undergoing that enable you to bond with your baby. Unfortunately, the changes to the structure of the brain are also suspected to make you more susceptible to mood changes (Barba-Müller, Craddock, Carmona, & Hoekzema, 2019). There are numerous risk factors that increase the likelihood of mood changes during and after pregnancy (Giardinelli et al., 2012; Ross, Steele, Goldfinger, & Strike, 2006).

## Activity:

Here is a list of common risk factors for Perinatal Mood and Anxiety Disorder (PMADs) listed by categories. As you read through them, ***circle any risk factors that you identify with***. This can be a helpful exercise to illuminate the various factors impacting your current mood and symptoms. This exercise will show you how complex these causes can be to your moods and how they can affect a wide range of women (adapted from Kleiman & Raskin, 2013).

| Environmental/Social: | Biological: | Psychological: |
|---|---|---|
| Multiple births (twins and more) | Previous PMAD | Prior pregnancy loss |
| Difficulty with breastfeeding | Prior history of mental illness | Young/teen mom or older mother |
| Separation from baby (baby in NICU) | Family history of mental illness | Perfectionist traits |
| Lack of social support | Infertility treatments | Unplanned/undesired pregnancy |
| Geographical isolation | Medical problems (i.e. thyroid) | Low self-esteem |
| Relationship problems | Breastfeeding weaning | History of trauma |
| Recent losses | Advanced maternal age | Unresolved grief over miscarriage or termination |
| Economic /life stressors | Re-starting birth control in postpartum period | Negative relationship with one's own mother |
| Recent moves/job changes | Decreased frequency of exercise | Negative self-image |
| Margarinalized communities (i.e. microaggressions, racism, etc.) | Pelvic floor pain/damage (perineal tearing at birth) | Traumatic birth experience |
| Single Parenting | Endometriosis, difficult periods | Difficult baby temperament (i.e. baby with cholic) |

**Adoption or surrogacy experience**

**History of PMDD/ PMS**

**Returning back to work**

**Pregnancy bedrest**

**Pregnancy complications (i.e. hyperemesis and pre-eclampsia)**

**Stress of pregnancy complications**

**What did you notice?** For example, how many risk factors did you circle? Were you surprised by your results? Do you tend to be more affected by environmental, biological or psychological factors? **Was there anything else interesting you learned about yourself?**

_____

_____

_____

## Important Takeaways

- After taking the screening questionnaires you may be better able to identify symptoms that you are experiencing right now. It can be helpful to determine what specifically you are feeling so that you can create a plan for feeling better.

- By identifying what you are feeling, and sharing it with one safe person, it can often be an empowering way to start fighting any internalized sense of shame or blame for these symptoms. You did not ask to feel this way, and you did not cause this!

- There are numerous risk factors for developing Perinatal Mood and Anxiety Disorders and mood changes. Environmental/social, biological and psychological factors can make you more at risk for these mood changes. This is not your fault!

**Part II**

# Building Tangible Skills to Help You Weather the Storm

# CHAPTER 5

## SLEEP AND SELF-CARE

### *TANGIBLE WAYS TO CLIMB OUT OF THE BLACK HOLE*

Bethany Warren, LCSW, PMH-C
Beth Creager Berger, Ph.D.

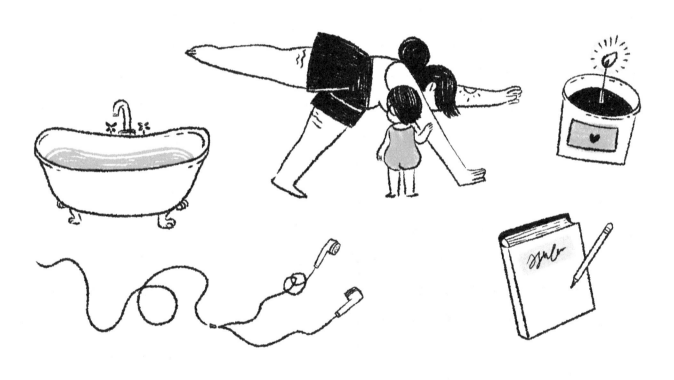

To love oneself is the beginning of a lifelong romance.

- *An Ideal Husband*, by Oscar Wilde

DOI: 10.4324/9781003144021-7

What is self-care? Self-care is what we do to take care of ourselves and to keep ourselves running, particularly when we have so many obligations and responsibilities in life. It is a way of soothing ourselves and taking care of our needs, both emotionally and physically. It's funny that self-care has become so trendy, and it is great that it has! As therapists, we love that self-care has become a topic that people are talking about so often in social media and in daily life because it makes it so accessible. However, people sometimes think of self-care as only grand gestures like getting massages or time away from home by themselves. These certainly count too, but it is also important to recognize the small things we do for our mental wellness and stability that fall under the umbrella of self-care too (especially during this season of your life as new parents!).

However, depending on how you were raised, and how self-care was modeled (or not, in some cases), this concept may be a difficult one, and wrought with guilt or shame. Perhaps you were raised in a culture where caring for others is really valued. This can be a complicated issue in becoming a parent and needing care, too. This chapter will help you find tangible ways of tending to yourself during this vulnerable time, no matter what your prior experience with self-care has been. Sometimes it's the small steps that help you feel better and the small victories that help you find your way back to yourself. Self-care activities can be practical and/or pleasurable and some are critical for functioning (like sleep or eating regularly).

**"Just surviving" level of self-care:** Much like a red stop light, which means "stop," we cannot move forward in life unless these basic self-needs have been met. It is important to recognize these activities as self-care too. Often we are not recognizing and giving ourselves credit for these foundation-securing activities, particularly when we are new parents. These might include **(put a checkmark next to any of the activities that you are doing on a daily basis)**:

- ☐ Showering

- ☐ Brushing my teeth

- ☐ Healthy eating and/or eating at regular intervals

- ☐ Regularly moving my body

- ☐ Wearing clean clothes

- ☐ Getting adequate sleep (i.e. sleeping between baby's feedings at night)

- ☐ Having and keeping a basic schedule for predictability and safety

- ☐ Spending time with my pets

- ☐ Communicating with my partner or with key people in my life

Can you see how some of these basic needs often fall by the wayside after having a baby? This is why if we only think of self-care as the big-ticket items, such as manicures and pedicures, we feel like we are failing when we cannot schedule those. And, by the time we do engage in some pleasurable activities, we are exhausted and cannot even enjoy ourselves fully. Attending to basic self-care is important to prevent feeling deprivation and chronic fatigue, particularly when you are already battling mood symptoms, such as depression or anxiety, which can be fatiguing themselves. The little stuff you are doing really counts! We need to give ourselves credit for accomplishing the basic things which are so important.

### Minute of Me (AKA M.O.M.):

- Stop whatever you're doing and just breathe. You're doing a great job and deserve a little micro-break. Pause and enjoy a good deep cleansing breath (or two). You've got this.

**"Making it work" level of self-care:** These are the important activities we can attend to once our basic needs are met and we are feeling more secure. Once our basic needs are being met, we can start attending to higher level self-care and becoming more efficient and productive. These are important but not vital, and often enhance our weekly routines. They can be especially helpful for new parents struggling with troublesome moods. These might include **(put a checkmark next to any of the activities that you are doing on a regular basis)**:

- ☐ Learning how to delegate some activities to others
- ☐ Setting boundaries (i.e. saying no to an event you don't want to go to)
- ☐ Implementing meditation or mindfulness practices
- ☐ Listening to music
- ☐ Creating shortcuts (i.e. ordering groceries online or having a meal delivery service one night a week)
- ☐ Reducing waste (immediately recycling junk mail rather than letting it pile up)
- ☐ Creating routines such as doing laundry once a week on a certain day
- ☐ Outsourcing and building your village: having some help in the house (family member, neighbor, friend, doula, mother's helper, nanny or housecleaner)

---

### Minute of Me (AKA M.O.M.):

- Take a minute and text a friend to remind yourself you're not alone.
- Or, take a moment to think about one thing on your "to do list" that you could delegate to somebody else. Suggestions might include offloading laundry this week or asking your partner to do a night feeding, if possible.
- You're not alone. You've got this.

---

**"Rocking it" level of self-care:** This level of our self-care is when we are able to do more of the pleasurable things for ourselves once our basic needs are met. These can also now include connecting with others because caring for others is best when it comes from a place of abundance of self, rather than when we're depleted and drawing on our own reserves. For most people this is a goal they work towards, not necessarily something that comes naturally (and with what you're currently experiencing with symptoms of a mood or anxiety disorder, you may not be here yet, and that's ok). This also can include **(put a checkmark next to any of the activities that you are doing)**:

- ☐ Social time with loved ones
- ☐ Date nights
- ☐ Self-pampering (Manicures/pedicures, haircuts, waxing, etc.)
- ☐ Catching up with a friend by phone
- ☐ Offering to chair a committee or volunteer for a project
- ☐ Reading/time alone
- ☐ Regular exercise

**Minute of Me (AKA M.O.M.):**

- Take a moment to plan a self-date over the next week that feels luxurious. Suggestions might be time with a friend, a facial appointment, alone time (gasp!), etc.
- You've got this.

## Activity:

**What are some of the fundamental self-care activities on your** *"Just surviving" level* **list that you are either currently doing, have previously done or want to do?**

_____
_____
_____
_____

**What are some of the important self-care activities on your** *"Making it work" level* **list that you are either currently doing, have previously done or want to do?**

_____
_____
_____
_____

**What are some of the pleasurable or nurturing self-care activities on your** *"Rocking it" level* **list that you are either currently doing, have previously done or want to do?**

_____
_____
_____
_____

**What one thing can you commit to add or change to each of your lists this week?**


**Just Surviving level:**
_____

When?
_____

How?
_____


**Making it Work level:**
_____

When?
_____

How?
_____


**Rocking it level:**
_____

When?
_____

How?
_____

**Minute of Me (AKA M.O.M.):**

- When did you last eat?

- It's common as a new parent to skip meals, grab snacks on the go, and feel underfed and hungry. This might make you feel shaky and tired, and worsen any mood symptoms you're already feeling.

- You are doing a great job of focusing on your baby's nutrition – this gets to be a moment of focusing on yours. Grab some nutritious, filling food the next time you have a moment.

## Identifying Deficits:

Doing the above activity may have been quite difficult, and it can be for a lot of new parents. It may feel like a lot is out of your control right now, right? Let's help you feel more in control by taking small steps. Identifying WHAT is overwhelming is a good start. What is keeping you from taking care of yourself?

As you went through the activity, did you find that you were lacking **support** in order to get your needs met? Did you find yourself struggling with **guilt** about putting yourself first? Are you lacking the **resources or financial means** in order to achieve some of the things you would like to do? Notice the themes we have just listed: ***support, guilt, means***. These are common barriers to self-care, but not insurmountable barriers.

## Activity:

**If any of these barriers resonate with you, please list them here:**

***Support:*** For example, "I don't have anyone to watch my baby yet," or "I'm alone all the time," or "none of my family lives nearby" or any other barriers around support that you're dealing with.

_____

_____

_____

***Guilt:*** For example: "I feel so guilty going back to work," or "I feel bad taking time to myself when I don't work," or "I don't deserve a break, I should be the one who takes care of my baby," or "I spent so much time and effort going through infertility treatment, I should always want to be with my baby now," or any other barriers around guilt that you're dealing with.

_____

_____

_____

***Means:*** For example, "I don't have money to pay for childcare," "I can't afford to pay for an exercise class for myself," "I really could use a sleep trainer but I don't think I can afford one," "I'm so tired but I can't afford to miss a day of work," or other barriers around means that you're dealing with.

_____

_____

_____

**So, what if I've hit a wall? Ideas for overcoming barriers:**

## Activity:

As you have thought of the self-care strategies you want to implement on a short-term and long-term basis and identified the deficits of support, guilt, and means, this is now an opportunity to think about HOW you might overcome any lingering barriers.

For example, you miss socializing and you have identified several barriers (*"all my friends work"*, *"no one will understand what I'm going through and I just don't have the energy to fake it"*, *"it still scares me to drive by myself with my baby"*).

Let's help you problem-solve how you might overcome these hurdles. This is a way to problem-solve and think through how you might address any barriers of taking care of yourself. **Check any that you would be willing to try**.

## Support

- ☐  *I don't have much support who live nearby but I've heard that new mom support groups are a good way to meet people. I'm going to look up one and attend this week.*

- ☐  *I miss my friends and even though I'm scared they might judge me for how I'm feeling, I will try to text a friend to reach out.*

- ☐  *I don't have anyone that I trust yet, but I really am craving some time away by myself. So in the meantime, I'm going to find a mommy and me exercise class to at least get a little of that part of my life back.*

- ☐  *I'm going to ask my neighbors for their babysitter's phone numbers for when I'm ready.*

- ☐  *I'm going to see if my neighbors are willing to do a childcare exchange with me.*

- ☐  *Other ideas include:* _____

- ☐  _____

## Guilt

- ☐  *I feel so guilty leaving my baby and I'm not ready to spend time alone yet. So, in the meantime, I'm going to try to find activities for myself that also include my baby until I feel ready to leave her with somebody.*

- ☐  *I feel guilty going back to work so I will talk to my girlfriend, who is a working mom, about that; I bet she will know what I'm going through.*

- ☐  *I feel so guilty about leaving my baby and taking time to myself, since I previously had a pregnancy loss. I feel like I should want to be a parent 24/7 now since I wanted this so badly, but I'm also so tired. While I'm still grieving and adjusting to new parenthood at the same time, I'll keep reaching out to my support who understands how complicated this is.*

- ☐  *I feel guilty about returning to work so I will think about what I can do to focus on bonding with my baby in the mornings and/or evenings, such as holding her for 5–10 minutes and talking to her or making sure I'm the one who does bath time.*

- ☐  *Because I'm a stay-at-home parent, I feel guilty using a babysitter. In the meantime, I will ask my partner or a family member to remind me that taking time to myself makes me a better mom.*

☐   *Other ideas include:* _____

_____

## Means

☐   *I don't have money to pay for an exercise class for myself so maybe I'll ask my neighbor to go on a walk with me.*

☐   *I don't have money to pay for childcare so I will make a list of family members, friends, and other people in my community that I would be willing to ask for help.*

☐   *I don't have money to hire a sleep trainer so I will look up some good books online and ask some other parents that I trust for some guidance.*

☐   *I'm so tired but I can't afford to miss a day of work so I'm going to work out a tag team system with my partner and/or family and friends to help me a few nights a week.*

☐   *If I am concerned about not being able to miss work, I also will check with Human Resources to inquire about my benefits and leave.*

☐   *Other ideas include:* _____

_____

*Andrea had a really traumatic birth experience and is now not only physically healing from her injuries, but she also can't seem to shake some pretty significant anxiety and nightmares. So when her well-meaning friend says to her "let's go get coffee", she wants to cry. How the hell is she supposed to shuffle out of the house wearing her big old diaper pad and accomplish that maneuver gracefully, not to mention find the mental strength to sit calmly in a coffee shop and focus on a social conversation? She desperately wants to be able to do that eventually but knows she's not even close to being able to socialize yet. Andrea's husband lovingly suggests that instead, her friend can bring them dinner, and maybe she will only stay a few minutes. That way, Andrea can see a friend and feel nurtured. Andrea loves that idea, and asks him to help her set that up since it seems too overwhelming to arrange anything right now.*

## Sleep As Self-Care:

Sleep is absolutely fundamental, isn't it? If you are not getting enough sleep (which is subjective and different to every parent), then everything is impacted: mood, patience, concentration, and certainly your ability to care for yourself. If you are not sleeping due to your mood or anxiety disorder, then everything can quickly snowball. Unfortunately, we expect all new parents to be tired. Even a new baby who is sleeping "well" disrupts the prior sleep routine a new parent was used to. Because new parents are typically so tired, it is a red flag if you cannot sleep when your baby is sleeping because you cannot shut down your thoughts. It is an indicator that you can use some help. A large percentage of our sessions with new parents are spent talking about sleep. Let's explore how sleep is for you and what you can do about it.

## Activity:

**Below, identify how many hours a night you are getting, on average, of sleep.** Some questions to ask yourself: How many times, typically, are you waking up?

Is the baby waking you up, or are your thoughts?

Are you able to fall asleep after feeding the baby? Or, is your body or your thoughts keeping you awake for a significant period of time?

Do you feel like your level of tiredness throughout the day is manageable (even if it's hard) as a new parent? Or, is it outside of your window of tolerance?

Are you able to nap sometimes during the day when the baby does (in other words, can you shut your thoughts down)?

## Sleep Hygiene

Much like the term "good hygiene" means you are regularly caring for your body's cleanliness, "sleep hygiene" is a term used to describe tips for maximizing your best sleep. One of the greatest contributors to mood symptoms is a lack of sleep. You might be laughing out loud at this because we know how tired you are. But better sleep is not fully out of your control.

Although a lack of sleep is not a direct cause of depression and anxiety symptoms, it does make you more susceptible to these emotions. When you are tired, it is more difficult to draw on coping skills that may normally serve you well. Because you may not have control of the *amount* of sleep you are getting currently in this stage of life, let's talk about different coping strategies to maximize the *quality* of sleep you are able to get right now. If getting more quality sleep is possible, it can help you manage your symptoms by allowing you to think more clearly. Below are some recommendations for getting your best sleep during your pregnancy or postpartum period:

1) **Stick to a sleep schedule as much as possible right now**. It may not be realistic to be rigid with a schedule given the season of life that you are in, but try to go to sleep around the same time every night. Being consistent reinforces your sleep–wake cycle and helps you fall asleep easier at night (this will get easier and easier as your baby gets older; doing the best you can is the key).

2) **Consider breaking up your night schedule to promote better sleep.** Depending on the age of your baby and the feeding method you're using, you and your partner might be able to split the night into two or more sections. The hope is for you to get at least a four-hour window of sleep, again depending if this is possible given how you're feeding your baby. Some couples split the night into two with one person doing the last feed of the night and one doing the early morning feeding, so that both can be "off duty" for a solid chunk of time. Others will trade off

entire nights so that only one parent is "on" a few nights a week. Single parents can benefit from family or friends staying over during the crucial early phase. See what might work for you, your baby's age, and your temperament.

3) **Be mindful of what you are eating and drinking**. Avoid caffeine in the afternoon and be mindful of limiting how much liquid you drink before bed so that your bladder is not waking you up in addition to your baby. Try not to go to bed either hungry or overfull.

4) **Establish a bedtime ritual**. Just like babies love bedtime rituals, we often crave them as well. When you use the same lotion for your baby after bath time, read and rock him in a dimmed room, etc., these calming activities tell him it's time to quiet down. Similarly, we can benefit from nightly rituals that tell our brains to wind down and prepare for sleep. This might include taking a warm shower, listening to calming music or a meditation app, and reading a book with dimmed lights.

5) **Create a comfortable bedroom space.** Create a room that is ideal for sleeping with darkened shades, a cooler temperature and one that is as quiet as possible.

6) **Move your body daily, if possible**. Exercising earlier in the day is even more preferable, especially when you are also exposed to outside sunshine or indoor bright lights. Even a brief gentle walk counts!

7) **Manage stress and stimulation before bed**. The two hours before bedtime can be considered your sacred time and a time to avoid bright screen time (TV, phone, computer) and stressful activities (homework, bill paying, conflictual conversations) if possible. This helps your brain wind down and prepare for sleeping.

8) **Journal about what you may be anxious about**. Write down these anxious thoughts to work on (examples to help you will be shown in Chapters 7 and 8). Or, buy a journal to work on when you experience anxious thoughts.

9) **Use meditation and other apps for relaxation**. There are many great apps and podcasts to help you wind down and meditate with a focus on sleep. See our resources chapter for some of our favorites. The options are limitless! Even a 10-minute meditation once you are in bed will help you tune into your body and regulate your breathing.

10) **If you cannot sleep, do not stay in bed for more than 30 minutes**. After 20–30 minutes get out of bed and read or relax but try not to engage in any stimulating activity, such as scrolling on your phone. When you start to feel tired, return to bed and try again but do not stay in bed awake for more than 20–30 minutes.

11) **Monitor alcohol intake**. Alcohol can disrupt sleep throughout the sleep cycle causing you to wake through the night (and alcohol is a depressant).

12) **Use professional help as needed**. If you find that your brain and/or body continue to keep you awake, please talk to a therapist, psychiatrist, or doctor (ideas are in our Resources Chapters). *There are many options to help you and you are not alone in this.*

## Activity:

**Of the things that we have just listed, what two or three things can you incorporate into your sleep routine starting tonight?**

_____

_____

_____

---

### Minute of Me (AKA M.O.M.):

- Take one minute as you are in bed with the lights off to practice a calming meditation to quiet your mind and body.

- You can use a meditation app to help (suggestions are in our Resources Chapter)

- The goal is not necessarily to fall asleep faster but for your body to learn how to relax and unwind at night. You've worked hard today!

---

_Good sleep is worth a million dollars, isn't it? Catarina would give anything to have good sleep again. She knew that sleep would be hard after having a baby, but she didn't know it would be THIS hard. When her daughter wakes up every few hours to eat throughout the night, that's hard enough, but at least that makes sense to her because that's what babies are supposed to do. What's harder to deal with is her own mind. After putting her baby back down, Catarina's brain is now fully awake and cycles through everything that could possibly go wrong in life. She sees all the horrible things that could happen to her baby, herself, and her spouse. Sometimes her mind even worries about things that don't even matter right now like thinking about when she will eventually go back to work! Catarina's therapist suggested she needed more "chunks" of sleep to allow for these more awake/restless times. So, she and her spouse now split the night in two: he takes the first half, she takes the second. While she still certainly wakes up when the baby cries and she hears her husband as he's feeding their baby, it helps knowing she's "off duty". She's also finding it easier to fall back asleep using a meditation app. For the first time in months, it seems like things are starting to turn a corner._

## Outsourcing as Self-Care (How to Get Yourself Some Help!)

How hard is it for you to ask others for help? It is for most people! It can be helpful to think of times of our life as seasons, and you may have previously been in a season of your life where you were capable of being able to care for others. But it is important for you to know that **this _is a season of your life of receiving care._** We frequently hear it in our practices "but I was always the one who looked out for my friends." "I've never been one to ask for help, it would be too hard." Often asking for help comes with negative beliefs about oneself such as "that means I'm weak", or even more simply "it's just hard to do".

It's hard to raise children alone and it is important to recognize that you are growing as a mother and can use all the help available. Some women may already have support around them through family and friends who instinctively know how to help. Other women may need to start building that help for themselves (even if they do have loved ones) and learn to outsource and build their village. Expanding your village is a way of practicing self-care. Remember, taking care of yourself ensures you will be able to take care of your baby with the best of you, not with what is left of you.

You can outsource by hiring help, ask trusted loved ones, or even get creative with shortcuts for help. **Check any that appeal to you**.

**Ideas for outsourcing include:**

☐ loved ones such as family, friends, or people from your community

☐ hiring professional help like postpartum doulas

☐ lactation consultants

☐ nannies

☐ sleep experts

☐ nutritional experts

☐ pelvic floor rehab specialists

☐ physical therapists

☐ physical trainers, etc.

**Ideas for what to ask for help from others include:**

☐ asking trusted family, friends, members from your religious community, neighbors, coworkers, etc., to participate in a meal train

☐ asking trusted family, friends, members from your religious community, neighbors, coworkers, etc., to come visit at times that work for you

☐ or asking trusted family, friends, members from your religious community, neighbors, coworkers, etc. to help you with tangible things that seem overwhelming, such as laundry, driving older kids places, etc.

**Ideas for shortcuts include:**

☐ ordering groceries online

☐ using tech help like a task completion app

☐ hiring house cleaners

☐ using meal delivery services, etc.

## SUNLIGHT EXPOSURE

Did you know that getting sunlight is a pretty easy way to boost your mood? Sunlight exposure can help regulate the production of Serotonin, a neurotransmitter responsible for the regulation of mood and Vitamin D, also thought to be responsible for mood (Berk et al., 2007). Serotonin also helps with the sleep/wake cycle and not enough sunlight can cause disruptions in sleep and major dips in mood. Have you ever heard of Seasonal Affective Disorder (SAD)? It can occur during the darker winter months where there are less bright hours of the day. SAD is thought to be at play during these months when people experience dips in their mood. (Graw et al., 1999). As you are likely aware, dips in mood can happen during the isolation that can naturally occur during the postpartum recovery time. Sunlight can help. Even if you aim for 10–15 minutes of sunlight exposure a day, that can be a great start. Try a brief walk to your mailbox with your baby, or sit in the sun with the baby monitor while your little one is inside napping. What other ways can you incorporate sunlight exposure at this time?

**Minute of Me (AKA M.O.M.):**

- The next time you can, take a moment to find some sunlight.

- Whether you rock your baby by a window, take a brief walk out to your mailbox, or sit on your balcony, how can you make sunlight a priority today?

- If this is not the season for light (or it is challenging to leave your space right now), how might you find some bright light inside today?

## Activity:

We have gone over a lot of self-care ideas and strategies now, and now you have an idea of various techniques that you could implement starting today (and some you could see yourself doing in the future). **As you start building your self-care list, what three (or more!) changes could you implement right now in order for you to thrive and keep going?**

Maybe you love the idea of incorporating more movement and want to start walking two to three days a week. Or, maybe you're going to work on your sleep hygiene by limiting the amount of social media scrolling you do before bed. What's it going to be for you?

_____

_____

_____

_____

### Rewards

Last but certainly not least, let's talk about how important it is to reward yourself. What you are doing is hard work. You may not be feeling well and are doing your best for both yourself and your baby. This is a good time to remind you that what you're feeling right now is temporary and will change. Because you might be in the thick of it right now, it's important to have positive reinforcement to help get you through. For example, if you are having a hard time with anxiety and you have been tending to isolate, please reward yourself every time you push yourself to get back out there and leave the house! Whether you stop and get your favorite coffee or listen to music to pump you up on the way, it's important that you are recognizing the effort you are making so you will want to do it again. Similarly, if you have been struggling with depression and low motivation and energy, give yourself breaks and pleasurable rewards at the end of any activity that takes effort. You deserve this.

**Some things that are rewarding for me are (examples are gifts for yourself, time to yourself, time with friends, a fancy coffee drink, pleasurable music or TV shows, or something you like to read):**

_____

_____

_____

## Important Takeaways:

- As a pregnant or new parent, there are some aspects of your sleep that are out of your control. Learning how to improve the sleep you are getting can be a game changer!

- Self-care is not always about self-pampering or having a lot of time to yourself. Learning how to interweave microbreaks and small time for yourself can make a world of difference right now.

- Figuring out any barriers for how to practice self-care will help you make small steps towards change.

- Getting even 10 minutes of sunlight exposure a day can positively impact your mood!

- Starting to build your village and expand your support network not only takes the load off your shoulders but also helps you feel less alone.

**CHAPTER 6**

# ATTACHMENT AND BONDING

## *CREATING A SECURE FOUNDATION WITH YOUR BABY WHILE IN THE MIDDLE OF YOUR STORM*

**Bethany Warren, LCSW, PMH-C**
**Beth Creager Berger, Ph.D.**

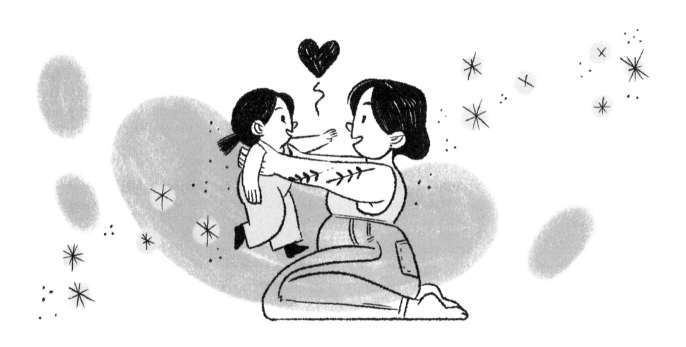

The very most profound thing we have to offer our own children is our own healing

- Anne Lamott

DOI: 10.4324/9781003144021-8

There is so much pressure to feel an ooey-gooey bond with your baby from day one, right? And if you're already feeling awful mood-wise, this pressure can make you feel even worse. Perhaps you do feel connected with your baby and everything else internally feels awful, or maybe you're struggling to find a connection with your baby. Perhaps you adopted your baby and are even more focused on promoting a secure bond with him. Or maybe, you had a difficult relationship with one or more of your own parents and are particularly mindful now about "getting this right". Regardless of your motivation, this is the chapter for you. We want to help give you ideas to promote the best connection between you and your baby and remind you that this is a judgment-free zone. We want you to know you are not alone.

*A close friend of ours had an experience with her first child where she did not feel connected to him after he was born. Her husband felt that the birth of their first child was the best day of his life at that point. To our friend, it probably did not even rank in the top five. Even though she knew he was her son, she felt he didn't look anything like her or her husband and had to remind herself he wasn't switched at birth. And yet, for whatever reason, this lack of connection did not bother her. She remembers saying "I'm sure you are mine so I will take care of you even though I really don't feel that connected to you." This was before the time anybody was ever talking about postpartum depression or perinatal mood disorders. For whatever reason, our friend had confidence that she would grow to love him and would eventually feel more connected to him with time. She felt equally disconnected to her next two babies, initially, as well, but knew that it would change.*

Our friend's experience is not uncommon. Other women, though, may feel guilt and shame and wonder: "What is wrong with me if I don't feel connected to my child?" or "Why don't I feel that instantaneous bond with my baby that I'm supposed to feel?" We are here to let you know that nothing is wrong with you and that your connection, if you are struggling, will come in time.

So let's talk about why attachment to your baby is important. Attachment between a parent and baby is critical and creates the foundation for much of the baby's life. One of the ways we learn how to care for ourselves is by modeling how we were initially cared for. Secure attachment with a child:

- enables them to imitate the parent and eventually build the crucial skill of empathy (Gopnik, Meltzoff & Kuhl, 2009).

- helps them learn to self-regulate through emotions.

- is reflected in their physiological state. When a baby is in sync with her parent, her security is reflected in a steady heartbeat and breathing and low stress hormone levels (Tronick, 1989; Tronick & Beeghly, 2011).

- helps them create what is called an internal locus of control - i.e. the ability to learn what makes them feel good or bad, how they can change how they feel about situations and have choices in their responses (Main, 1996).

Secure attachment with your baby helps them set the tone for their relationships with others by teaching them what they can expect from interactions and experiences. It is a two-way feedback loop; the baby reads your cues as you read theirs. A secure attachment between a parent and baby is essential for wellbeing.

The great news is that the majority of mothers do well in managing this by being what researchers call a "**good enough mother**", versus a "perfect parent", recognizing it's impossible to respond to all of a baby's cues at all times. Basic things like practicing eye contact and talking to your baby are important in creating safety for him and helping him feel safe, connected to you, and secure. Research has shown that even down to the way that mothers hold their babies helps lay the groundwork for the baby's sense of self and a sense of identity (Winnicott, 1971).

**Hey, How're You Doing?**

- This may trigger feelings of shame right now if you're not feeling a strong bond yet with your baby.

- Let us reassure you that impacts from a lack of strong attachment can be undone.

- Step by step, your attachment will grow. You're working on it, keep reading.

**If your baby could thank you for something you are doing well for them right now, what would that be? (Check all that apply.)**

☐ Feeding them

☐ Holding them when they cry

☐ Bathing them sometimes

☐ Changing their diapers

☐ Looking in their eyes sometimes

☐ Talking to them

☐ Doing your best right now

**Anything else you can think of?**

_____

**The overlap between attachment and mood symptoms:**

So how do perinatal mood symptoms come in? Unfortunately depression, anxiety, or trauma during the perinatal period can impact attachment with the baby in some mothers. It makes sense, right? If you're in survival mode, it can be challenging for some to also care for another little being, much less feel warm and connected to them. It's like you're already treading water, trying to stay afloat, and somebody hands you a baby. It would be really challenging to keep swimming AND be nurturing to the baby, right? We write about this very gently, recognizing that you are likely already anxious, wanting to do your best and already feeling incredibly guilty. First let us remind you that your mood and emotions are NOT YOUR FAULT. You have picked up this workbook which is a great start and shows that you recognize something is off and are wanting to change it. Second, not every mother's mood or anxiety disorder _does_ impact bonding with her baby, but if it does, it can be addressed, and it is important that we talk about this frankly.

**Hey, How're You Doing?**

- This chapter will help in promoting a bond with your baby and also remind you that you are not alone in what you are experiencing.

- Despite feeling depressed, when women work on attachment building skills, bonding improves (Jung, Short, Letourneau & Andrews, 2007).

- New research shows that birth related PTSD does not impact bonding (Radoš et al., 2020).

Women whose depression goes untreated can struggle with bonding and connecting with their babies. They often feel less confident with parenting, read and talk less frequently to their babies, and even feel more disengaged (McLearn, Minkovitz, Strobino, Marks & Hou, 2006). However, what we do see continually in our practices is that women who address their Perinatal Mood and Anxiety symptoms have a positive impact on their connection with their babies. It is inspiring to watch women start to feel better themselves, and then see a positive impact on their bonding with their babies. Attachment *and* self-soothing can be learned skills. It is important for you to work on attachment in addition to your own self-care.

Maybe you're worried about the attachment you have with your baby. Maybe you're worried that you're not bonding with your baby. Maybe you worked really hard to have your baby, going through years of fertility treatments or you experienced pregnancy losses, and now are extra worried that your bond with your baby isn't "good enough" or where it should be. Maybe you've heard that attachment is super important and it IS important. But here's the secret truth about attachment . . . it takes time. Bonding with your baby is a process and you can do this. We're going to show you how.

You may be wondering how to foster attachment even when you don't feel it. Here are some small ideas you can start incorporating today:

## Activity:

Below are some ideas to help promote attachment and connection with your baby. Whether you are dealing with Perinatal Mood and Anxiety symptoms or not, every mother/child can benefit from a secure connection and strengthened bonds. **Enjoy choosing one or more from the list to practice**. Just spending one minute practicing any of these moments of connection is sufficient and a great start.

\_\_\_**Practice looking into your baby's eyes and smiling**. This is not a hard one for all mothers, but can be difficult for moms who are feeling really depressed, so this can be a "fake it until you make it" moment. Notice what happens as you breathe and just smile when your baby is calm. Practice tuning in to your baby's face.

\_\_\_**Talk to your baby**. It truly does not matter what you are talking about because your baby *loves* the sound of your voice (and has been hearing it throughout your entire pregnancy!). If you do not know what to talk about, practice describing what you are doing, what you are thinking, what you are planning for the day, etc. This promotes connection with your baby as your baby wants to hear *you* no matter what you're saying.

\_\_\_\_**Wear your baby** (in a sling, wrap, etc.) Your baby will love the connection next to your chest and this will help promote bonding and attachment (and also frees your arms up, an added bonus!)

\_\_\_\_**Practice "skin to skin" time** after bath or diaper change, placing your baby on your chest for a few minutes or whatever is tolerable, and talking to her softly. Notice her breathing and your own, and see if you can just notice the smell of her, the softness of her skin, becoming in tune with her body against yours.

\_\_\_\_**Read to your baby**. Remember, your baby loves hearing your voice. Whether you're reading a recipe to him, a blog you find interesting, or an actual baby book, your baby will love hearing your voice. Notice whether your baby prefers a more soothing voice, a sing-song voice (even if you feel silly), and how it may depend on his mood.

\_\_\_\_**Practice baby massage.** Whether you use a soothing lotion after bath time, or massage over clothes while you and your baby are connecting on the floor, practice getting to know your baby, talking softly, and looking into your baby's eyes. There are some great videos that can teach you actual techniques if you would like, or you can just go with your instincts, if you would rather.

\_\_\_\_**Build in quiet time interactions**. When your child is calm (yes, even a child with colic), use the calm moments to mirror her calm. If her eyes are averted, notice this cue as "I need a break" and practice sitting in the quiet. If she looks at you, notice this cue as "I'm checking in" and speak quietly and warmly to her, quieting again when she looks away. This is a great exercise to practice tuning in and getting in sync with each other's rhythms.

\_\_\_\_**Watch for signs that your baby wants to play and engage**. If he is smiling, kicking, and inter-active, you can get down on his level, talk with him, and play using toys and animated language. This is a great time to smile and mirror his expressions (notice as he grows that he will mirror your expressions back!)

\_\_\_\_**Also watch for signs when your baby wants to take breaks and is overstimulated**. She may keep her eyes averted, be more fussy, or show other signs. Please be reassured, you may miss these cues sometimes, this is part of becoming in sync and learning your baby's cues!

**Of the above suggestions listed, what are some bonding activities that you can start?** Also list when a good time is for you to engage in these activities (e.g. just after feeding or before I put her to sleep). Give yourself credit for accomplishing some of these interactions. An idea would be to post these on the fridge and check them off when you try one.

**The positive news:**

The good news is that not all parents who have mood and anxiety symptoms during the perinatal period will have an impaired bond with their baby. In fact, in our clinical practices, we frequently see deeply depressed and anxious parents who are struggling to get through the day and feeling awful themselves but are still capable of deeply loving their babies. This may be what kept them from seeking help initially, saying "I haven't been feeling like myself, but I love my baby, I thought depression meant I wasn't connected to my baby at all".

But even if that connection is not fully there yet, and you are feeling guilt as a result, *you can do something about it*. Some mothers may not yet feel that deep bond with their baby because bonding is truly a process that can take time to develop. Yet, they are able to tend to their baby's basic needs like feeding, changing, and holding their baby. Even if they feel like they are "going through the motions".

Parenthood is hard no matter what, especially that first year. It is so much harder when you are struggling with mood and/or anxiety symptoms. This is a tough job and you are doing it. As you work on healing yourself and bonding with your baby, both things will improve, and this chapter will help you feel more connected to your infant.

## Activity:

Whether you are dealing with mood swings, depression, or intrusive anxious thoughts (or all of it!), you are still doing your very best to take care of your baby even if you are not where you would like to be yet as a parent.

**Even if you feel like you are just going through the motions or faking it sometimes, or maybe you feel guilty about how you are feeling, what is one (or more) thing that you think you are doing to tend to your baby's needs?**

_____

_____

_____

These things you just named ARE what connects with your baby. Tending to some of your baby's needs is a way for you to connect even if you don't feel that strong bond yet.

---

### Hey, How're You Doing?

- A reminder that bonding is a process that takes time.

- Parents bond with their children at different ages; it is common for one parent to enjoy the infancy stage, for example, whereas another might not feel bonded with their child until the toddler stage when they have more interaction and feedback.

- Treatment for depressive symptoms can improve the feeling of being bonded to your infant (Mulcahy, Reay, Wilkinson, et al., 2010).

---

Let's face it, depression and anxiety are so hard. It is exhausting to deal with a million intrusive thoughts a day or the hypervigilance of anxiety, feeling like you are constantly warding off doom and catastrophe. It is so tiring to fight the lack of motivation, low energy, irritability, and brain fog of depression. It is fatiguing to go through the cycle of mood swings of bipolar disorder, feeling so high and out of control, then so low and sluggish. And it is certainly exhausting to have been through a traumatic experience and still feel like you are in "trauma time" and not safe even though the event has passed. So, of course mood can have an impact on attachment with a baby even when it is unintentional.

Parents can sometimes not even know they are out of tune with their babies and miss relevant cues if they are so preoccupied with their own mental health or symptoms. Disconnection can happen if you continually reach out to your baby for engagement and it feels like you are unable to soothe or connect with him (van der Kolk, 2015). Anyone who has had a colicky baby certainly knows how stressful this situation can be! It can be easy to internalize this as "I'm a bad mother" or project this on the baby by thinking "my baby is difficult" or "my baby doesn't like me" if there becomes a pattern of difficult interactions. If you find yourself frustrated easily or disconnected, _you are not alone!_ This is where support groups can be helpful to receive validation from other parents, and support and coaching from a therapist can help you gain insight and skills to connect with your baby as well as help to heal from your own symptoms. _You are not alone and it's important to get help._

_Alex feels like a fraud. If one more person says to her "isn't this the most magical time?" she just might scream. She thought she was supposed to feel some magical connection to her baby the moment he was born but that didn't happen. She felt numb and disconnected, almost as if she was watching it all take_ *place to somebody else. She keeps expecting it to happen, whatever "it" is, but she honestly does not feel much toward her baby. Sure, she is capable of doing everything she needs to in order to take care of him: she bathes, rocks, changes, and even breastfeeds him. If anyone watched her, they might say she is a good mother, but she just does not feel the warm "ooey-gooey" feelings she is "supposed to" feel, and that makes Alex feel like a monster. When she looks into her son's eyes she feels like she is failing him. And sometimes she even avoids his gaze. Surely he deserves better than her. It's like living with a stranger. She is trying her best, but not really understanding what he is trying to say, and it feels like he does not really understand her either. It is easier to hand him off to others and let other people take care of him, especially when he is crying; it is such a helpless feeling not knowing what he needs. This all just feels so shameful and she cannot tell anyone, because surely nobody would understand.*

*Carrie also does not feel very connected to her daughter. She had a traumatic and scary birth and was so focused on everything happening around her that it makes some sense to her that bonding with her daughter unfortunately took a backseat to safety and survival. She is beginning to feel more capable of taking care of her baby over time. It feels less scary now and less like she might break her, though she still sometimes would prefer someone else do the baby care when she has intrusive scary thoughts, and honestly, sometimes taking care of the baby feels like a chore. Carrie doubts herself constantly, feeling like a bad mother and wanting to feel more connected with her daughter, but deep down has hope that her bond with her will grow with time. She is noticing that things are changing, she is starting to learn about her baby, like the difference between her cries, and finds that her baby responds to her differently than she does to other people. Even though it is really hard right now, Carrie has some confidence that things will change and get better.*

You've got this. Bonding is a process and it takes time to develop a connection with your baby and learn his cues. While your own symptoms may be taking some of your attention and energy, you are addressing them and that is admirable. We thank you on behalf of your baby. This is so important.

## Important Takeaways

- Whether you are struggling with mood symptoms, or are just growing into your new role as a parent, it is important to promote a growing secure attachment with your baby.

- You are already doing a great job, and there are simple ways of connecting with your baby that can help you both feel more secure and attached.

- Secure attachment with your infant can help them learn amazing skills such as empathy, self-regulation, and self-control.

- Bonding with your baby comes with time.

CHAPTER 7

# MOM GUILT AND OTHER MIND BATTLES

## *HOW TO MANAGE YOUR THOUGHTS, MOODS, AND BEHAVIORS USING COGNITIVE BEHAVIORAL SKILLS*

Bethany Warren, LCSW, PMH-C
Beth Creager Berger, Ph.D.

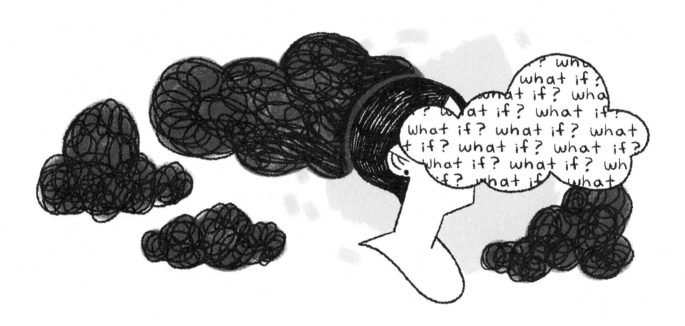

We are shaped by our thoughts, we become what we think

- Gautama the Buddha

DOI: 10.4324/9781003144021-9

Do you ever have thoughts that everyone is a better parent than you? Do you feel like you are a failure as a mom or a bad mom? Do you worry your child will meltdown if you take her out and then people will judge you? We all struggle with negative thoughts, and disruptive thoughts are really common during the postpartum period. Quite frankly, these thoughts are common throughout parenthood as well. We're here to help you learn how to identify and manage your thoughts so they don't negatively impact your mood.

This is a rich chapter with many activities to help you learn skills to manage your moods, so take your time. This is a great chapter to pick up and put down, and not to be digested in one sitting (particularly if you're a tired new parent!).

Our thoughts, moods, and behaviors are all related. For example, our thoughts can influence how we feel, which then guides our behaviors. A cycle can then continue. This chapter draws from inspirational Cognitive Behavioral Therapy authors who have paved the way in creating these concepts (Burns & Beck, 1978; Beck, Rush, Shaw, & Emery, 1979; Burns, 1980; Greenberger & Padesky, 1995).

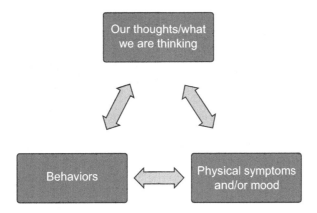

*Emma is feeling exhausted, depressed, overwhelmed, and has low energy. She thinks to herself: "this new mom thing is so hard but everyone else seems to be having such a joyful, easy time with the transition". When she is on social media or out at the playground, it seems all the other moms look like they have it all together. She wonders what is wrong with her and wonders why it is so difficult for her. She thinks everyone must have figured out by now that she is not a good mom so she stops going to her play group and slowly stops socializing.*

### Emma's cycle looks like this:

*Thoughts:* "What's wrong with me? Everyone seems to be a better mom than me. They all have it so together and I feel like I can't even get it together. They must think I'm a terrible mom."

*Physiologic (body) symptoms*: lethargy, decreased energy

*Mood symptoms:* sadness, guilt, shame

*Behavior:* avoiding play groups and social situations

*Continued Thoughts:* "I saw a photo of my friends all together on social media. They all seem so happy. They don't want to be with me because I am such a downer."

*Worsening Physiologic (body) symptoms:* lower energy, lethargic

*Worsening Mood symptoms:* increased sadness, feelings of loneliness, decreased motivation

*Unhelpful Behavior:* avoids social situations *and* continues to isolate further

As you can see from Emma's example, negative thoughts can often "feed" emotions and body sensations which then lead to unhelpful behaviors. These can often cause thoughts to become stronger and the cycle continues to spiral downward.

## What is Cognitive Behavioral Therapy?

Cognitive Behavioral Therapy (CBT) is a type of treatment that disrupts the negative thoughts–feelings–behaviors cycle. In this chapter, we are drawing from the CBT model to help you identify any thoughts that are impacting your current mood symptoms, and help you see how these thoughts have guided your behavior. Research has shown CBT to be effective in treating depressive and anxiety symptoms in about eight to twelve sessions with a therapist (Clark et al., 2015). We are specifically teaching you these skills here because we find CBT useful in our own practices, and there is specific evidence that CBT is effective in treating Perinatal Mood and Anxiety Disorders (PMADs) (Sockol, 2015; Wenzel & Kleiman, 2014). This chapter introduces you to the concept of CBT and encourages you to make small adjustments so that you can change the cycle of depression and anxiety. If you keep working on these skills, you will notice improvement in the way you think about things and the way that you feel!

---

### Did You Know?

- CBT is effective in addressing mood and anxiety disorders, including Perinatal Mood and Anxiety symptoms (Buck, Zekri, Nguyen, & Ogar, 2019).

- Research has shown CBT apps to be effective in improving postnatal depression (Jannati, Mazhari, & Ahmadian, 2020). Look for app suggestions in the Resources Chapter.

- 60% of people who go through Cognitive Behavioral Therapy with a therapist for the treatment of depression or anxiety get better (DiMauro et al., 2013; Dobson, 1989; Huang et al., 2018).

---

## Changing Behavior

In the same way that thoughts, feelings and behaviors can create a cycle of worsening moods, it is possible to change one of those components, for example changing your behavior, and this will affect the rest of the cycle. It can be quite difficult to talk yourself out of your thoughts initially because those thoughts **feel** so real and they may be thoughts that you have struggled with for a long time. In fact, resorting to that negative thought may even have become a habit.

Changing the behavior that does not serve you is a good place to start which will then have a positive impact on the rest of the cycle (our thoughts and mood). For example if Emma starts with making small adjustments to her behavior, despite feeling unmotivated, the whole cycle will change.

*Initial Thoughts:* "What's wrong with me? Everyone seems to be a better mom than me. They all have it so together and I feel like I'm a mess. They must think I'm a terrible mom."

*Physiologic/body symptoms:* lethargy, decreased energy

*Mood symptoms:* sadness, guilt, shame

*Purposeful Behavior:* (Even though it's really hard), walk with my neighbors

*New Thought:* "Although I feel like I don't have it together, the other women seemed ok having me around and it was good to not be by myself."

*Improved Physiologic/body symptoms:* a little less lethargic; a little more energy

*Improved Mood symptoms:* more hopeful, happier, more confident

*Changed Behavior:* Walking with my neighbors more often

*Continued New Thought:* "I feel connected to others and I feel a little bit better than I did before."

These small changes can positively affect your mood. Although it will take time to feel like you're back to yourself, small changes can begin to take the edge off your mood and help you toward the path of feeling good again.

Emma's old cycle:

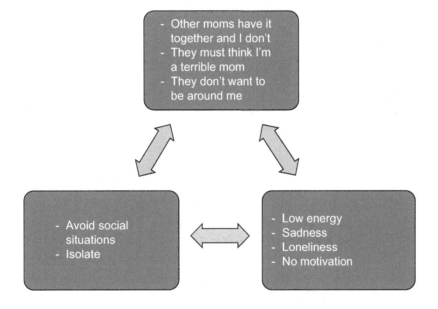

Emma's new cycle:

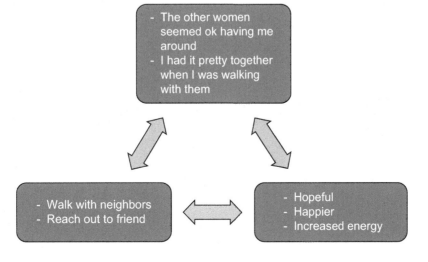

## Activity:

**List any of your behaviors that you are currently concerned about or have changed since becoming pregnant or having your baby.** These might be unhealthy coping mechanisms like avoidance of situations that make you anxious or isolating from others due to your lack of energy. Additional examples might be avoiding alone time with your baby, distancing from your partner, overeating to soothe yourself, etc.

_____

_____

_____

_____

**What small changes might you make to the behaviors you noted above? What might make these more healthy or adaptive for you right now?** An example might be if you are avoiding your friends due to fears that they will judge you, that you will reach out to one friend who you feel can be safe. By texting her, you have made one small change. We know it's hard, but by taking this first step, you've made a decision to land your plane, so to speak.

_____

_____

_____

_____

## PLEASURABLE ACTIVITIES

Often when people are feeling depressed or anxious they no longer seem to enjoy activities that they used to find pleasurable. They avoid activities that they used to like. However, isolation and avoidance tends to continue the cycle of depression and anxiety. Instead, it can be helpful to take small steps and begin to re-engage in activities that you may enjoy. You may not enjoy the activity as fully as you used to but the idea is to try and engage in some pleasurable activities more than you are currently.

## Activity:

**Make a list of some short/quick activities that you have enjoyed in the past that you can do when the baby is napping, when you have help, or when your baby is playing near you.** Ideas include reading a book, gardening, listening to a podcast, watching a tv show you like, or walking with a friend. Suggestions can also include ideas you came up with from Chapter 5: Self-Care.

_____

_____

_____

_____

**Now, make a list of some longer activities that you have enjoyed in the past.** Ideas include going to the movies, meeting a friend for coffee, doing a craft or hobby, or attending a yoga or exercise class.

_____

_____

_____

_____

**Choose one or two of these activities you could engage in during this week.**

_____

_____

List two days and times you will try to engage in the shorter pleasurable activity, for example, during baby's first nap of the morning:

| Day | Time | Activity |
|-----|------|----------|
| 1.  |      |          |
| 2.  |      |          |

List one to two days and times that you will try to engage in one of the longer pleasurable activities:

| Day | Time | Activity |
|-----|------|----------|
| 1.  |      |          |
| 2.  |      |          |

(It may be helpful to schedule a reminder for these in your calendar.)

## SOCIALIZING

Are you lonely? Do you miss your friends and talking with other adults? Is it unsatisfying when you talk to your baby about all the things you have planned for the day and she doesn't share your enthusiasm? Babies are great at a lot of things but they're terrible conversationalists. Often, new moms feel isolated with few other adult friends. It is not uncommon for new moms to feel lonely, bored, and even unproductive. With these feelings often comes feelings of grief and sadness. Planning time to get together with a friend or family member can help decrease these feelings, particularly when you are struggling with mood symptoms.

**List some friends or family that you can make plans with:**

_____

_____

_____

_____

**List some activities you can do with these companions** (these don't have to be huge activities; even just sitting and talking, or walking with your baby helps you find connection):

_____

_____

_____

_____

## Did You Know?

- If this was a tough section for you, you're not alone!

- Many new moms struggle with isolation and feeling disconnected from their old friends.

- Chapter 9 will help give you ideas for reconnecting with your support network and building a stronger village. The Resources Chapter will also give you some ideas for new parent support groups and other ways of connecting with new parents.

## Physical (Body) Changes

### Physical Exercise

Moms are the queens of multitasking, and we are not going to make you stop. In fact, you can make multitasking work for you during this season of your life. When you don't have a lot of spare time or energy, it can be helpful to interweave small changes in ways that feel feasible to your current lifestyle. Some additional behavioral changes you can also make that will positively impact your physical and mood symptoms are exercise, meditation, and relaxation. We will review meditation and relaxation more in depth in Chapter 10, but we thought it was useful to mention here so you can start thinking of tangible behavioral changes you can make now.

Exercise produces endorphins that help people feel better. When you're used to exercising and stop due to pregnancy or having a baby, your body may miss the endorphins it was used to and you then may have feelings of lethargy, anxiety, and/or sadness.

Research suggests that for every 25–30 minutes of elevated heart rate through exercise, depression and anxiety symptoms decrease (Dimeo et al., 2001). Even starting out with a ten-minute walk a day, or doing leg lifts while brushing your teeth is moving your body again. This can take the edge off some of those negative symptoms and perhaps give you a little more motivation or energy to continue to engage in activities that make you feel good.

## Activity:

**If you are cleared by your doctor or midwife to do so, write down one to three times this week that you can exercise** (even a short walk is a great way of moving your body!):

| Day of week | Type of Exercise | Length of time |
|---|---|---|
| _____ | _____ | _____ |
| _____ | _____ | _____ |
| _____ | _____ | _____ |
| _____ | _____ | _____ |

### A Review:

- Thoughts, moods, and behaviors are all interrelated.
- A change in any one of these will then change the cycle.
- One of the easiest parts of this cycle to change are your behaviors.
- Behaviors you have within your control are engaging in pleasurable activities, socializing, and physical exercise.

## Negative Thoughts

It sucks to feel like a bad parent. It's hard to have a running narrative of self-blame and negative self-talk. And, it's draining to have a hamster wheel running of anxious thoughts, right? Mood symptoms are often fueled by negative thoughts about oneself. These thoughts often fire automatically when we are not feeling good about ourselves.

Some common negative thoughts of parents are **(check any you have experienced)**:

- ☐ *I'm not good enough*
- ☐ *I'm a bad parent*
- ☐ *People don't like to be around me*
- ☐ *I can't do anything right*
- ☐ *I'm a failure*
- ☐ *I'm broken*
- ☐ *I'm unlovable*
- ☐ *I can't soothe my baby*
- ☐ *I'm a bad mom for going back to work, I'm neglecting my baby*
- ☐ *Working moms have it so good, what's wrong with me that I get so bored and resentful during the day?*
- ☐ *My baby must not like me*

☐ *Everyone else is doing better at this than I am*

☐ *This will never change*

☐ *If I leave the house, I won't be able to handle it*

☐ *Another thought I'm having:* _____

The way we talk to ourselves can be so harsh, right? We would NEVER talk to a friend that way, particularly another mom friend that is struggling. And yet, why do we say these things to ourselves, and how can we learn self-compassion?

Instead of trying to talk yourself out of the thought, it can be useful to first learn how to identify when you are speaking to yourself negatively. It is like you've been listening to a radio station for a long time that has been saying terrible things about yourself, so much so that you end up believing them. We want you to learn how to change the channel. For example, if you are saying to yourself "I'm a horrible mom", it can be important to identify that this is a defeatist thought. Essentially your brain is lying to you, telling you that you are a horrible mom. Identifying the false narrative is the first step in learning how to change the channel.

## Activity Part I:

**For one week, keep a log of when you are feeling down or anxious. Identify the situation at the time that precedes your negative mood and then identify what you are thinking.**

Example:

| Mood | Situation | Sad or anxious thought |
|------|-----------|------------------------|
| *sad* | *yelled at my two year-old* | *I am a terrible mother.* |
| | | |
| | | |
| | | |
| | | |
| | | |
| | | |

This is a great time to take a pause and focus on just this exercise for about one week. You might need to add a separate page for adding any additional negative thoughts you catch. After learning to catch negative thoughts, we will guide you on how to look at those thoughts in a different, more empowering way in the activity parts II and III.

## SHAME AND GUILT

Shame in particular can get in the way of thinking rationally and it can get in the way of asking for help. Shame can be humiliating and distressing. For parents suffering from Perinatal Mood and Anxiety symptoms, the shame is often caused by a misperceived sense of being in the wrong. For example: "What is wrong with me?", "Everyone else is so happy", or "I must be a bad mom."

*Maya had three children under the age of six. She was never diagnosed with a PMAD. When her youngest child was a year old, she tearfully informed her husband that she realized that she had suffered from depression symptoms over the last year starting after her last baby was born. Maya's husband, who was usually supportive, was surprised. What symptoms did she have that he missed? He hadn't seen her tearful or struggling to take care of the children or return to work. Maya recounted the past year and all of the times she told her husband and children she was going to nurse the baby in her room. Truthfully, she admitted, although she would nurse the baby for 10–15 minutes, she would then hide in the room and read to avoid being needed by her husband or other children. One year later, Maya cried, describing the shame she felt for avoiding her family during those times. She described feeling inadequate as a result and like she was a bad mother for not being able to handle everything. Maya had felt she needed someone's permission to take time for herself, and had felt shame for sneaking in that time.*

What makes us hesitant to take time to ourselves? It is a common theme we see in our practices. Whether we're working outside of the home or stay at home mothers, women need to give themselves permission to take care of themselves without feeling guilt and shame. New moms often feel like they have to do it all, and without support. But the standard that new moms compare themselves to is often unattainable which breeds feelings of inadequacy. And feelings of inadequacy breed shame. Women often feel that they have to "do it all" or else they feel that they are not succeeding. The age of social media serves to exacerbate this phenomenon of comparing ourselves to others and feeling as if we are coming up short. "Not good enough," is a negative thought we see in new moms. The shame these negative thoughts create only serves to perpetuate the cycle of negative moods like depression and anxiety.

## Challenging the truth of your thoughts:

You may be saying "but my negative thoughts feel soooo real". You may be able to find some thread of evidence to support these thoughts which is why they feel so real. However, although at the time, these thoughts "feel" very real, they are not 100% rational and it is important to start looking at why these thoughts are not true. What would a friend say to you if you shared this thought with her? How would you respond to a friend with a similar thought? How do you change the thought so it feels true to you but is not so negative? The answer is to start focusing on why this thought is not true.

*Brie feels like a terrible mom. She knows she's doing this whole "mom thing" wrong and feels such shame anytime she sees her mom friends online. Their social media posts are the cutest and they're so active and creative with their kids! She has a hard time mustering the energy to do anything but the basics, and she can't help but wonder where all these "super moms" get their energy and creativity. When she finally shared this with one of her friends, the friend laughed and admitted she felt similarly. Her friend admitted she only posts the filtered, "good" posts about herself, and leaves out all of the times she's crying or a mess. She reassured Brie that she's not alone and that every mom struggles at times. She also pointed out that Brie is actually a great mom. She loves watching Brie cuddle her daughter, and admires how she is so vigilant about protecting her. Brie never would have known. Her friend helped her see that **she was comparing her insides to someone else's outsides**. Everyone has their "terrible mom" moments, but that doesn't make you a terrible mom. In fact, maybe they're just "normal mom" moments.*

You are doing your best, and by comparing how you are feeling to how others around you appear to be doing, you are comparing apples and oranges.

## Activity Part II:

Now that you have identified thoughts that may affect your mood, let's look at what makes these thoughts true for you and what may make them not true. And then, with this new perspective, we will look at healthier ways to view yourself. It can be useful to "play detective" and look for the evidence both for and against a thought.

For example:

| Defeatist / Negative Thought | What Makes It True | What Makes It Not True |
| --- | --- | --- |
| I am a terrible mother | I yelled at my 2-year-old and made him cry. | My children are usually happy to be with me. |
| | I don't enjoy motherhood sometimes. | I am feeding and taking care of my children. |
| | All the other moms seem calmer and happier than me. | My partner complimented me on my hard work with my family. |

Looking at your thoughts this way can be really difficult. **Take a few days to write down your defeatist thoughts and then look at what makes it true and what makes it not true.** If you have difficulty finding reasons the thought is not true, ask your therapist, partner, friend, or family if they can provide insight for you.

**Defeatist/Negative Thought**          **What Makes It True**          **What Makes It Not True**

_____

_____

_____

_____

_____

## Activity Part III:

Let's help you change the channel on your radio station. This is where all your work comes together. Now that you have a healthier way of seeing the defeatist thought, let's try and change the thought in a way that is less defeatist and more realistic.

In order to view your thoughts in a healthier way, it is ok to acknowledge some of what initially made the defeatist thought believable to you while also looking at what makes that defeatist thought not true.

For example:

*Although I sometimes lose patience with my children, I take care of their needs. I show them love and they seem to be generally happy.*

**After identifying a common, negative thought, ask yourself "what is another way to look at this?"** Write down your new, rewritten and adaptive thought for yourself (an example is given above). Notice how we've used a thought that is true, including the part that brings distress (losing patience) and the more realistic and balanced perspective (taking care of their needs, showing them love and seeing their happiness).

Although, _____, I _____

_____

_____

_____

_____

This may be hard. Keep after it! When you find yourself feeling sad or anxious, try catching your defeatist thought. And then see if you can look at the thought in a more realistic way. This takes time and practice and is much more beneficial if you can write the thoughts down on paper or on your phone or computer. The important part is that you write down the defeatist thought and then get to a place where you can develop a more realistic perspective. Learn how to listen to what's playing on the radio station and then change it!

## Important Takeaways

- Our thoughts, moods, and behaviors are all related. For example, our thoughts can influence how we feel, which then guides our behaviors.

- Behaviors are often the easiest of all of the parts of this cycle to change, and seemingly the ones most immediately within your control.

- Exercise, meditation, and relaxation are behaviors that can help change the negative cycle.

- Identifying how you speak to yourself (i.e. your negative, defeatist thoughts) is the first step in learning how to change your thoughts to more balanced, healthy ones.

# CHAPTER 8

# MANAGE AWFUL THOUGHTS

## NAME YOUR DRAGON TO SLAY YOUR DRAGON

Bethany Warren, LCSW, PMH-C
Beth Creager Berger, Ph.D.

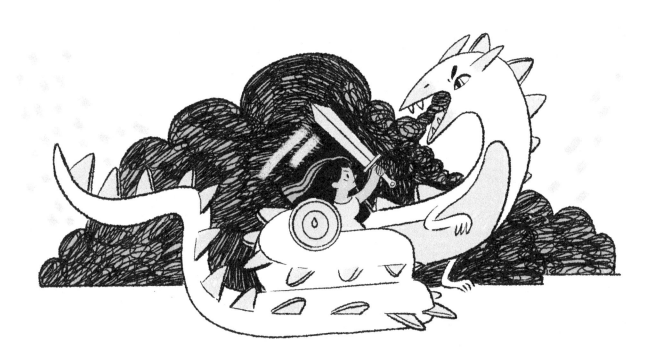

I am not afraid of storms, for I am learning how to sail my ship.

- *Little Women*, by Louisa May Alcott

DOI: 10.4324/9781003144021-10

EVERY parent has disturbing thoughts. Most have pictured dropping their babies at some point or something similarly distressing. And most parents recognize these thoughts as brief, passing, irrational thoughts. However, some people experience these scary thoughts on a repetitive loop (these are called obsessive thoughts) and will find ways to manage and control the distress from these thoughts. But the ways they sometimes manage the distress may eventually become unhealthy or unhelpful (these are called compulsive behaviors).

*Nahla is so freaked out that her baby is going to stop breathing at night, so she wakes up constantly to go check on him. She sometimes doesn't even fall back asleep and instead just constantly watches the monitor and will run back into his room if she thinks she doesn't hear anything. She feels like a zombie now, she's barely getting any sleep, and yet she's unable to sleep well. She's just so scared with the obsessive repetitive thought "my baby is going to stop breathing" she can almost hear it playing on a loop over and over. Unless someone else is vigilantly watching him, she feels unable to relax.*

Parents may avoid certain situations entirely, do compulsive behaviors such as cleaning to manage fears of germs, completely avoid distressing situations, or check locks repetitively to ensure safety. Some parents experience the obsessive scary thoughts without the accompanying behavior, but regardless, feel equally as distressed and helpless.

---

**Did You Know?**

- More than 90% of ALL mothers report having scary thoughts at some point (Kleiman, 2019)!
- Upwards of 40% of moms with anxiety or depression report they also have intrusive and unwanted images that pop into their mind (Zimbaldi et al., 2009).

---

Do you remember how in the previous chapter we went over how to identify automatic thoughts? Distorted thoughts often drive our emotions negatively and we often act maladaptively as a result. Hopefully you now have had a chance to think about some of the common automatic thoughts you are experiencing as a new parent and are considering some ways to make some small changes to the behaviors stemming from these thoughts.

Remember this cycle from Chapter 7?

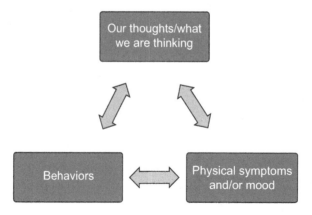

So what do you do when these thoughts you are having are super scary and intrusive? We recognize that there is a big difference between thoughts of self-blame like "I'm a bad mom" and more intrusive images like actually picturing something awful happening to your baby, particularly if the image involves your participation (i.e. causing harm to yourself or your baby).

We have purposefully chosen not to trigger you by giving you too many horrific, specific examples of some of the obsessive scary thoughts that we have heard throughout our years in practice. Instead, we hope that it helps you to hear about general themes of intrusive thoughts and images women often experience during the perinatal period so that you know you are not abnormal (and certainly know you are not alone!). **Check the ones that you can relate to experiencing:**

**Themes of thoughts/images:**

- ☐ General worry
- ☐ Germs and contamination
- ☐ Images or feelings of failure, loss, defectiveness
- ☐ Vivid illness, death or injury scenes pertaining to yourself or the baby
- ☐ Worries about your baby's caregivers
- ☐ Humiliating actions or mistakes
- ☐ Sexual thoughts
- ☐ Current events or stories seen in the media
- ☐ Worry about fidelity of spouse
- ☐ Body sensations
- ☐ Worrying about worry

Let us reassure you that whatever you are thinking will not rattle us. No matter how awful, visceral, and triggering your thoughts or images are, they are just that: thoughts, and you are not responsible for them. Let us say that again. **You are not responsible for your thoughts. Thoughts do not equal intention.** What you ARE responsible for is what you do with the thoughts you are having. By reading this chapter, or going to therapy, or telling your provider, you are taking initiative (and can learn another way of managing those thoughts). We recognize how hard this can be and you are taking an important first step.

We know it is very difficult to talk about your thoughts. In fact, in our clinical practices, we are typically the ones that have to initiate this conversation because most parents are scared that if they admit what they have been thinking or seeing that we would call the authorities on them! This is an important time to remind you again that **thoughts do not equal intentions**. Obsessive and scary thoughts are not the same as psychotic beliefs, hallucinations, or a desire to want to hurt anyone. The fact you feel distress about them is a good sign, funny enough, because it is a great indicator that you do not have a desire or intention to harm anyone. Psychotic thoughts, on the other hand, tend to be consistent with the person's worldview, and people do not try to fight these thoughts. They instead hold strongly to these thoughts, believing them to be true.

### Did You Know?

- Your intrusive thoughts do not mean that you intend to act on them.
- Thoughts do not equal intention.
- Obsessive thoughts are not the same as psychotic delusional beliefs or hallucinations.

## THE PARADOXICAL EFFECT

You may have noticed something really frustrating about your thoughts. The harder you try to fight them or control them, the more "sticky" they seem to be, right? The harder you try to not think about the intrusive, distressing images, the more they seem to linger and cause disturbance. This is what is considered a "paradoxical effect". It doesn't work when you are anxious and someone tells you to "just calm down", right? Nor does it work when you try this with yourself; telling yourself NOT to think about something or to "just calm down" only seems to give your brain the idea that this thought or image is actually distressing and should be focused on more.

For example, if we tell you NOT to think about tacos, not to think about the last time you had tacos, not to think about your favorite type of tacos, or to picture tacos, or how tacos smell, how much are you picturing tacos right now? It does not work to try to force ourselves to be calm, stop thinking about something, or let something go. So no wonder this has been so hard for you. And also, who else is now craving tacos? We sure are.

## SO, WHAT CAN I DO ABOUT MY THOUGHTS?

The skills you learned in the prior chapter about the thoughts–emotions–behaviors triangle are still relevant here and are transferable skills even if your distress level is high.

*Amira pictures herself dropping her baby every time she carries her baby up or down the stairs. She can see it so vividly it feels like it is actually happening, and sometimes she becomes so panicked she feels her heart racing and will sit down on the stairs for several minutes. It has gotten so bad that she has been avoiding the stairs with her baby lately. She has been making excuses to cover it up like asking her husband to grab something upstairs for her while she is downstairs, or asking him to carry the baby up to bed "while I just do one more thing and I'll join you in a sec!". She feels so ashamed of the thoughts and she worries it means she might actually drop her son. She wonders, "What kind of mother would do that?" Even the thoughts themselves bring a sense of panic even when she is nowhere near the stairs. When that happens, Amira doesn't trust herself to hold her baby for a while, even if he is crying, which feels like torture to her. In fact, all of this feels like torture!*

As you remember from the last chapter, identifying the thought–feeling–behavior cycle is so crucial. Notice how Amira is distressed because she believes she might actually drop the baby as she has imagined.

### Amira's cycle looks like this:

*Thought:* "*I'm going to drop my baby when I carry him up the stairs.*"

*Physiologic (body) symptoms:* panicked, heart racing

*Mood symptoms:* anxiety, panic, guilt, shame

*Behavior:* avoiding the stairs, avoiding holding the baby

Are there any small, realistic behavioral changes that Amira could do to address this difficult situation? Ideas could include telling her husband why she has been avoidant of the stairs, and with his help (depending on their relationship), ask for him to walk with her as she carries the baby up the stairs. Amira could also hold the baby and just step on her first stair, breathing deeply and giving herself some positive self-talk and encouragement.

**Amira's new cycle, implementing this new behavior change would then look like this:**

*Old Thought:* *"I'm going to drop my baby when I carry him up the stairs."*

*Physiologic (body) symptoms:* panicked, heart racing

*Mood symptoms:* anxiety, panic, guilt, shame

*Behavior:* avoiding the stairs, avoiding holding the baby

*New Thought:* "With my husband's help, I might feel a bit safer to walk up the stairs with the baby, even though I'm scared."

*Physiologic (body) symptoms:* still anxious, heart racing

*New mood symptoms:* hopeful, feeling more empowered and safer, yet still anxious

*New behavior:* After asking her husband for support, walks up the stairs holding the baby with his help, practicing her slow breathing as she does.

Little by little, practicing this with time, Amira felt more comfortable and confident.

Unfortunately, avoidance just strengthens our belief that the situation is distressing and we cannot tolerate it. Small and more frequent exposures to the situation brings the distress down over time.

*If this feels too overwhelming to do on your own, this is where working with a therapist is crucial. You are not alone in this! Ideas for finding a therapist are at the back of the workbook under "Resources" and it is important to find one with a specialty in Perinatal Mental Health AND obsessive thoughts and compulsive behaviors.*

## Activity

If you are having scary thoughts, it can be helpful to just name them. Name your dragon to slay your dragon. Not naming your thoughts gives them more power. Remember, you are not your thoughts, and thoughts do not equal intention. **Write down your current thoughts or intrusive images you might be experiencing** (or what feels safe or comfortable to write down). Examples of themes of thoughts are on page 2 of this chapter:

_____
_____
_____
_____
_____
_____

**How do these thoughts make you feel? What emotions do you notice when these thoughts or images come up? (Check any that apply.)**

☐  Anxious
☐  Sad
☐  Guilty
☐  Ashamed
☐  Frustrated
☐  Irritable
☐  Resentful
☐  Terrified
☐  Hopeless
☐  Other_____

Sometimes identifying the frequency of your thoughts can be helpful not only in being real with yourself in how bad this is for you, but also can be helpful if you do decide to go see a therapist or psychiatrist – this is good information to relay to them. Additionally, identifying a pattern in which the thoughts seem to be occurring at a particular time of day or during a particular activity can be helpful.

**How often are you having these thoughts a day (roughly)?** (For example, at least five times an hour)

_____
_____

**Is there a time of day in which the thoughts are more likely?** (For example, they seem to be worse at night, or first thing in the morning as you are waking up)

_____
_____
_____

**How are you managing these thoughts or images with your behaviors?** (i.e. avoiding the situation, hiding objects that are a part of your thoughts in case you don't trust yourself, repetitively checking or cleaning, handing the baby off to others, isolating from seeing specific people or going outside, etc.)

_____

_____

_____

_____

_____

_____

_____

And this is the most important part: **do you have any ideas of what small behavioral step(s) you could or would want to do based on what you wrote above?** For example, if you wrote that you have been avoiding going outside entirely, what small steps might you recognize you could take towards that goal with some support? Or, if you're compulsively checking your baby throughout the night, what support can you seek to address this, such as talking to your partner or a new moms support group about your fears and getting a different perspective? Or, if you have been compulsively searching medical illnesses on the internet, perhaps set aside one time per week for one hour a day to search the internet and gradually reduce the frequency of time you spend searching medical illnesses.

_____

_____

_____

_____

_____

_____

_____

## Relabel and reattribute your thoughts

There are several treatment methods that aim to manage scary thoughts and/or the accompanying compulsive behavior. One way is to **relabel and reattribute the thoughts** (Schwartz, 2016). You can think of obsessive thoughts like undesirable buses that are going by you on the street. As a scary thought pops up, name it as an obsessive or intrusive thought, and watch it go by just like you would a gross, broken-down bus that you choose not to get on. "Ugh, there's that awful thought of me dropping the baby", and with time and practice, it will likely dissipate. Then, by reattributing it as an obsessive thought, and naming the underlying emotion, you are taking the power out of it: "ugh, there's that awful thought, it is distressing but doesn't mean it is real". By renaming it as an obsessive thought, you are reattributing it as something not real, even though it **feels** real. This then will help you **refocus** your energy on what you can control, like holding on to the railing as you carry your baby downstairs. You're now learning how to fight your dragon, so to speak.

Practice now relabeling and reattributing one of your thoughts. **Take one of your above-named thoughts or intrusive images, and relabel it as an obsessive or awful thought and not a truth.** For example: my obsessive thought is _____ and even though it feels real, it's just a thought.

_____

_____

_____

_____

_____

Exposure and Response Prevention (ERP) is a type of cognitive behavioral approach which is commonly used to address obsessions and compulsions as well. The therapist helps the client slowly reduce the level of distress by exposing them to their fears bit by bit, while adding in relaxing techniques to manage the feeling of fear.

---

**Did You Know?**

- There are things that you can do to manage your awful and intrusive thoughts and accompanying, unhelpful behaviors.

- The Schwartz four-step method is a treatment option to help decrease the frequency and intensity of obsessive thoughts.

- Exposure and response prevention (ERP) can also be a useful therapy to help decrease the frequency and severity of distress caused by scary thoughts and compulsive behaviors.

---

We have gone over some ways to manage obsessive thoughts and compulsive behavior but we want to say here that working with a therapist who is specifically trained in these treatment methods can be important in helping you find full success. This is hard work to do on your own and additional support can be useful with this matter. This workbook can be helpful at giving some basic ideas and helping you identify some core themes of what you are struggling with, but for deeper work, please see our Resources chapter.

## IMPORTANT TAKEAWAYS

- Having scary thoughts as a new mother is very common, in fact more than 90% of new moms report having them at some point!

- You are not responsible for your thoughts. Thoughts do not equal intention. (Even if they are scary, violent, or about your baby).

- If your thoughts are becoming repetitive, on a loop, these are called obsessive thoughts.

- The paradoxical effect means the harder you try to not think about the intrusive, distressing images, the more they seem to intensify and cause disturbance.

- Learning to name and reattribute your thoughts can be a small, but powerful change for your thoughts instead.

# CHAPTER 9

# ROLE CHANGES, SUPPORT, AND COMMUNICATION

## *STRENGTHEN YOUR VILLAGE*

**Bethany Warren, LCSW, PMH-C**
**Beth Creager Berger, Ph.D.**

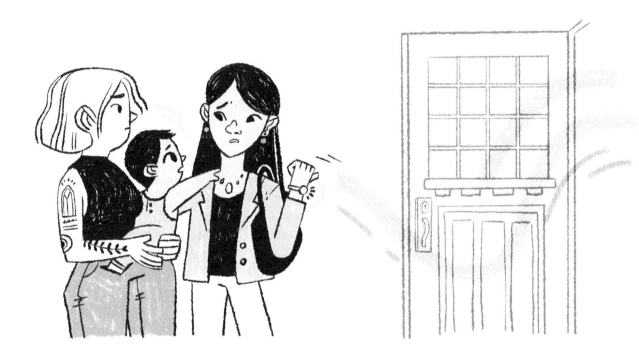

In times of stress, the best thing we can do for each other is to listen with our ears and our hearts
and to be assured that our questions are just as
important as our answers.

- Fred Rogers

DOI: 10.4324/9781003144021-11

There is no bigger change in life than becoming a mother. Becoming a parent has often come after years of dreaming about this next stage, reading and preparing and endlessly fantasizing about it. We often forget that giving birth to your baby also means that you are also essentially giving birth to yourself as a mother and that your new identity takes time to develop. For many, this abrupt shift into motherhood can be difficult to navigate, particularly when additionally struggling with a worsening mood. In our clinical practices, we often have clients share deep feelings of grief during this time, because in missing their old lives and their prior identities, they express a sense of profound sadness with this life change. While you may love your baby and have wanted this new change in your life, it may also be an incredibly difficult adjustment; both things are not mutually exclusive.

To add to the adjustment to motherhood, your new identity, and your life as it is now, you may also be grieving the ideal birth experience you had hoped for, how you thought you would feel, and what you had hoped parenthood would be. We often hear from our clients a sense of grief as they mourn the birth experience they thought they would have. This is even more the case if they had a traumatic birth experience and are then grieving the birth experience they had, coupled with the traumatic mood symptoms they might now be facing. We hear from many of our clients things like "I thought this would be so much easier" or "I thought this would be such a happier time". It is important to know this is a very common part of adjusting to motherhood, growing into your own identity and adjusting to what IS versus what you thought parenthood would be. It's already hard enough to adjust to motherhood, but then when mood symptoms are layered on top, it can become an overwhelming time! This can be a time of eventually learning "grudging acceptance" of what is, thereby allowing yourself to experience, and possibly grieve, what you ARE feeling. This will help you to not feel so stuck.

*Sarah finds that this is a season of "ands". She loves her baby AND misses her old life so much. She loves her son, AND really misses the freedoms she used to have. She feels really tied down now with such a rigid feeding schedule AND yet, she loves the closeness they feel when she feeds him. She hates how weepy she gets and how out of control her emotions feel and she misses the time where she felt like she was more solid emotionally. She gets scared when she wonders if she'll ever get herself back because she feels so different from her old life. She thinks of how capable she used to feel at work, how funny she used to be around her friends, and how she and her husband used to have a pretty good marriage. It seems like all they do is snip at each other now. She hates having to ask him for help because he seems to get so defensive, and it feels weird to be constantly having to remind him to do some really basic things. She misses her old life and her old marriage. And, deep down, while she loves her baby, and can't imagine life without him, sometimes she wonders with guilt if motherhood was a mistake.*

Within this chapter, we have drawn on the ideas of Interpersonal Psychotherapy, an effective psychotherapy particularly useful for PMADs (Spinelli, 2017). By reviewing what has recently changed for you (the various role transitions you have experienced as a new parent), you can better address what support you have currently and what needs you still have in building your "village." We will also review **how** to reach out for help, because asking for help is already so difficult and the way we talk to others shapes so many of our interactions.

## Role Changes

Not only are you not feeling like yourself, but you may be engaging with those around you in new ways, too. If you have a partner, part of this time of adjustment that can be especially difficult is the change in both you and your partner's roles and how you engage with each other.

You likely interacted in certain ways before the baby came and now this may have shifted and possibly has even changed dramatically. This can be a tough time on a relationship! Perhaps you were both used to being fairly independent. You likely didn't have to ask for your basic needs to be met (i.e. sleep, food, reassurance you are doing a good job, etc.). Or, perhaps without even speaking about it, you were used to the division of chores in your house.

---

### Did You Know?

- This can be a hard time for most couples to navigate.

- Upwards of 67% of couples report marital dissatisfaction after having a baby (Gottman & Gottman, 2007).

- In other words, you're not alone!

---

For example, maybe one of you did more of the cooking and the other always took out the trash. That may have changed now with the addition of your new baby.

These small changes can actually have a large impact on the ways that we interact with each other, and particularly so when we are sleep deprived, less patient, and struggling with depression and/or anxiety symptoms! You may be mourning the loss of being independent, feeling smart and capable in your career, and are now having to ask for a lot of help. You may feel resentment about having to ask for things that you think your partner should intuitively "just understand" but he or she may not. You may also now be grieving or adjusting to a significant change (or loss) of sexual intimacy.

If you are a single parent, you may notice these role changes even more significantly. You have a lot on your plate, and being a solo parent can be really overwhelming. All decisions fall on you, and you have even less time to yourself. It may be hard to ask for help. Being vulnerable may feel abnormal to you if you are used to being independent.

## Activity

**As you read the section above and start thinking about all the changes you have experienced in becoming a new parent, what stands out to you? Below, list some of the largest changes you have noticed** (i.e. loss or change in career, loss of independence, a change in communication patterns with your partner, feeling like your friends don't understand you now, excitement about a new phase of life, feeling of responsibility with taking care of someone else, etc.):

_____

_____

_____

_____

_____

We give you a lot of credit for doing that exercise above and recognize that even naming some of these changes, particularly some of the changes in the roles in your relationship, are really hard. Facing this is important, though, and we commend you for taking this step!

**Now pay attention to some of your strengths as you notice these changes. During this time of change, what are you noticing that you are capable of?**

Examples of strengths or abilities might be (**put a checkmark next to the ones that resonate with you or add some of your own below**):

☐  I do love my baby even though this is hard right now

☐  I'm trying to stick to a schedule

☐  I am taking care of baby's basic needs

☐  I'm learning from my mistakes

☐  I'm parenting differently than how I was parented

☐  I am using some of the good parenting skills I learned from my own parents

☐  I'm doing the best I can

☐  I'm loving and connected to my baby

☐  I'm patient at times

☐  I'm figuring this out

☐  I'm learning how to ask for help

☐  I'm taking a shower (sometimes)

☐  I'm leaving the house (sometimes)

☐  I'm figuring out how to exercise or move my body

☐  I'm learning how to eat throughout the day

☐  I've returned to work and I am contributing financially and emotionally to my family

☐  I've returned to work and I am learning how to manage my new schedule

☐  As a stay at home parent, I'm learning what I need in order to manage my new role

☐  As a stay at home parent, I'm proud of what I contribute to my family

☐  I'm a good friend

☐   Other

_____

_____

_____

Remember, no one expects you to have checked all the boxes. The purpose of this is for you to reflect on some of your strengths.

You are going through a major life transition. With all of the changes you have noted above, this is one of the largest changes of your entire life. It can be quite difficult, and with difficult things, we often can learn a lot about ourselves as a result. **What are some positive things you are learning from this experience of becoming a new parent?** Perhaps you are learning that you are capable of harder things than you ever thought possible, or that you can still take care of your baby despite really struggling. Maybe you are really having a hard time but you are learning that you like being a mom at times. Or, even if you aren't currently enjoying this stage of life, you are hopeful it will change.

_____

_____

_____

It is ok if that section was harder than the previous one particularly if you are still in the middle of your struggle with your symptoms. This is where working with a professional therapist might be helpful in assisting you in setting goals and pointing out what you ARE doing well. We suggest also asking your partner or a close loved one, if this feels safe, what they think you are doing well as a mother. If you skipped this section because it was difficult, we encourage you to come back to it during some point in your healing because it is really important.

## Interpersonal Inventory

The other thing that often drastically changes after having a baby is your support network. We often hear from our clients their disappointment and even grief about their relationships changing. While it is common for relationships to shift after you have had a baby, we know it can be quite unsettling as well. Perhaps you were really close to a set of friends who no longer reach out to you as much or cannot relate to your new life. Or, perhaps you feel like the old you is gone. This can be particularly true when also experiencing mental health issues; how isolating it is to be fighting this battle when you don't even feel like yourself! It takes effort to reach out, and many women struggle with feeling ashamed when admitting to others what they are going through.

That stigma of mental illness coupled with some negative thoughts like "nobody knows what I'm going through" can really amplify the feelings of isolation and loneliness. The next exercise can be a helpful reality check to take stock of the support you DO have.

## Activity

Below, notice the two circles. This is called an Interpersonal Inventory, taken from the work of Interpersonal Psychotherapy (Stuart & Robinson, 2012). Consider that you are the dot at the center of the innermost circle. **Now place a handful of your support people throughout the rest of the circles, thinking of the proximity to you as an indication of your emotional closeness, the tangible support they provide you, how much trust you have in them, etc.**

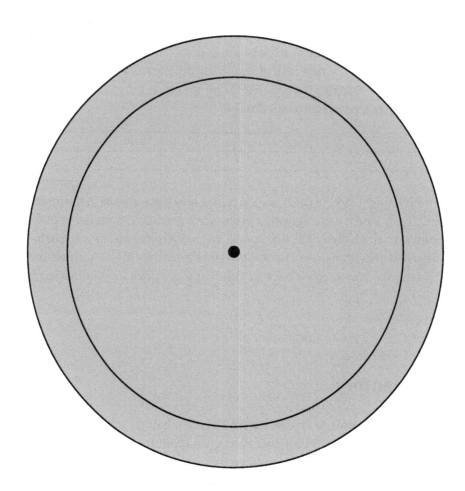

**Now consider the placement of the people.**

- Who is the closest to you, and what function do they provide in your life?

_____

_____

_____

- Who is missing from your inventory that used to be there (i.e. what has changed with your inventory over time)?

_____

_____

_____

- Were there any surprises as you were placing people within your inventory? Did you find that someone was closer to you than you'd imagined, or vice versa?

_____

_____

_____

- What was this experience like emotionally? Any sadness or regret about any of your support? Any relief about realizing you have the support you need in certain areas?

_____

_____

_____

- Now this is one of the most crucial aspects: where are the gaps in your support? For example, you might notice you need more tangible, hands-on support from people who can come into your house to help with the baby. Or, perhaps you noticed you need more emotional support.

_____

_____

_____

- And finally, what do you have within your bandwidth right now to address? This might mean that you notice a close relationship has drifted apart but you could really use this person in your life right now. Do you have the energy to invest back in that relationship by reaching out right now?

_____

_____

_____

If you noticed there are people missing or outside of your inner circle that you would like to move closer but are not knowing how to do so, let's move to the next section to learn how to reach out in an effective way.

## Effective Communication Skills

### (i.e. How to Effectively Ask for Our Needs in a Way So That Our Loved Ones Can Actually Hear And Respond to Us)

So often in our work, we observe our clients reaching out to their support, trying to express their needs. Yet, unfortunately the **way** they ask results in their partner or loved ones either responding in an unhelpful way, ignoring their request completely, or not meeting their needs. This can become an ugly feedback loop when a new mom withdraws from her loved one, saying "I don't get help anyway", the loved one feels helpless and may say something like "I don't know what to do to help you", or "I can never do anything right" and resentment and anger build in the relationship. Does that feedback loop look at all familiar to you?

_Gabby feels so hopeless about her relationship. It seems like ever since they've had their daughter, nothing goes smoothly between her and her wife. It used to be pretty easy between them, but now when she asks her wife to help, she seems to get really defensive, saying things like "you always tell me I'm doing everything wrong". Gabby isn't sure where things went south, but it's gotten to the point where now she just wants_ *to do everything for the baby by herself, but because she's feeling so anxious, that feels virtually impossible and really overwhelming. But when she asks for help, it's hard to watch her wife handle the baby and it's like her heart is in her throat the whole time. She can't help but hover, give her advice, and ask her to be more gentle, but apparently the way she is doing it makes her wife really mad. It feels like she is stuck between a rock and a hard place, because she needs the help but can't say anything without making her wife upset.*

The way we communicate with each other, even when we are calm, can sometimes make things worse. And this is particularly true when we are stressed out and sleep deprived! Even a passive aggressive response can evoke a really hostile response from our partner. Instead, if we ask for our needs specifically and directly (rather than vaguely and aggressively), we can yield a more beneficial response. This will ultimately make it easier on both of you, because both of you are tired and need things to go smoother.

---

### Did You Know?

- A good communication skill that is helpful in expressing your needs directly is using an "I" statement (adapted from Markman, Floyd, Stanley, & Lewis, 1986).

- The basic premise is:

  "I felt _____ (emotion) when _____ (objective description of event) happened, and what I need instead is _____ (direct expression of need).

- An example is: "I feel overwhelmed when I am pumping and do both prep and clean up by myself. Could you help me by changing a diaper while I'm setting up the pump, and clean the pump parts while I'm storing the milk? It would be so helpful and take a huge load off my plate. I'd get back to sleep sooner, too, an added bonus. How does that sound?"

## Activity

This can be challenging to do but is really important right now as you think about improving the support you DO have (i.e. your partner, family members, friends) and think about the quality of your communication. If you are willing to sit with this exercise for a bit with honesty, it can be tremendously helpful in getting your needs met.

## Patterns of Communication:

**What patterns of communication are you noticing in your primary relationship?** (i.e. when I reach out, I am often angry and he responds defensively, or, when I am anxious, I'm quick to shut down and get quiet and she thinks I'm mad at her so she pulls away, etc.)

_____
_____
_____
_____

## How I Ask for Help:

**How do you tend to ask for help?** (i.e. I just figure he should know what I need, or I let my resentment build until I'm so frustrated I explode and tell her how angry I am that she's been ignoring all the household duties and I have to do everything, or I am really detailed with saying exactly what I need and why, etc.)

_____
_____
_____
_____
_____

**When I ask for help, my partner (or family member) tends to respond by...**

_____
_____
_____

That may have been hard to note some communication patterns that you may not be proud of, or may feel pretty hopeless about. Writing them down and noticing them is a great start and we're so proud of you! Helping you learn what the issues are is truly the first step to changing things. And again, you're not alone!

## Am I Jumping to Conclusions?

It is really common that when you are sleep deprived, frazzled, and just doing your best, you can be more snappy at your loved ones. It is also pretty normal to jump to conclusions and make a lot of assumptions about what they are thinking based on minimal information. For example, how often does it feel personal if your partner doesn't pick up after him or herself? You might be telling yourself "he just doesn't care about me! I've told him a million times how aggravating it is to pick up his laundry when he's a grown adult; it's like he doesn't even care about how exhausted I am". Or, if you don't hear back from a family member when you've reached out, you might feel rejected and have your feelings hurt. It's understandable, you're going through a lot right now!

Sometimes, though, we will have jumped to conclusions without having all of the information. And it can be helpful to check in to let our loved one know what we're thinking, what we think they're thinking, and see if it's accurate. Here's a sample script to "check it out" with them:

"When I see your socks on the ground after I've asked you to pick them up, I feel like you just don't care about how exhausted I am and that my requests aren't important. But I'm wondering if there's another explanation. Can you help me understand?"

Or

"When I texted you and didn't hear back from you, I worried maybe I overshared about my depression that I've been going through and I felt so embarrassed. But I'm wondering if there might be something else going on?"

**Can you identify times when you tend to jump to conclusions with any of your loved ones?**

_____

_____

_____

**What situations would you be willing to practice "checking it out" with them?**

_____

_____

_____

## Optimizing Communication

We don't expect you to have all of the answers on this next part, in fact, this can often be really difficult for most people, and can be helpful to work with a therapist on identifying and changing patterns of communication. Remember the earlier statistic about how 67% of couples report marital dissatisfaction after having a baby (Gottman & Gottman, 2007)? Hopefully this reassures you that communication difficulties are quite common when becoming parents and experiencing the major shift in roles.

## How Clear Am I?

How clear do you think you are when you communicate? (For example, do you ask for specific help or do you imply what you need, getting frustrated when vague requests are not understood?)

_____

_____

_____

## Are We Choosing the Optimal Times to Talk?

What times do you typically approach your partner with your needs? Do you think you both are choosing the best time to approach each other with your needs? (i.e. when both of you are calm, not distracted, and able to commit to the conversation)

_____

_____

_____

## Activity

**Even if you don't have the answer on what to do yet, can you think about what is** *not* **working in your communication?**

☐  I am not direct with speaking up about my needs

☐  I expect my partner to know what I need (mind reading)

☐  I am defensive when my partner tries to tell me something is wrong

☐  We do not talk much except about the baby or our kids or things that need to get done

☐  We are rude to each other (name calling, criticize each other)

☐  We talk about issues that bother us in the heat of the moment (versus waiting to be calmer to talk about hot topics or issues that bother us)

☐  We stop talking to each other if we are upset

**Other Problem Areas of Communication:**

_____

_____

_____

_____

As you did the exercises above, what stands out for you? Are you in a space to address this right now? Do you have the means, time, or energy to address this in your relationship? The answer might be "no" given everything you are dealing with in addition to your mood. Realistically, though, it can be helpful to just know that it is common that communication is frequently affected when one partner is impacted by mental health issues. If you are not in a space to go to couples therapy, a communication workshop, or even address this in your own individual therapy, we will leave you with this question to ponder:

## Activity

**How can I ask for help more effectively?** (Ideas might be using an "I" statement, choosing a more optimal time to ask for my needs, try not to blame, be respectful in communication, being more direct/specific, etc.)

_____

_____

_____

_____

## Important Takeaways

- It's very normal to grieve the loss of your "old self" even if you are very happy to be a mother.

- These changes in your new identity can impact the relationship with your partner, how you view yourself, and how you communicate.

- This can be an important time to evaluate who is in your support team so that you can better get your needs met.

- Learning how to ask for your needs directly and communicate effectively saves valuable time and can improve the relationships you have.

# CHAPTER 10

# MINDFULNESS, MEDITATION, AND RELAXATION

## *HOW TO QUIET THE STORM WITHIN*

**Bethany Warren, LCSW, PMH-C**
**Beth Creager Berger, Ph.D.**

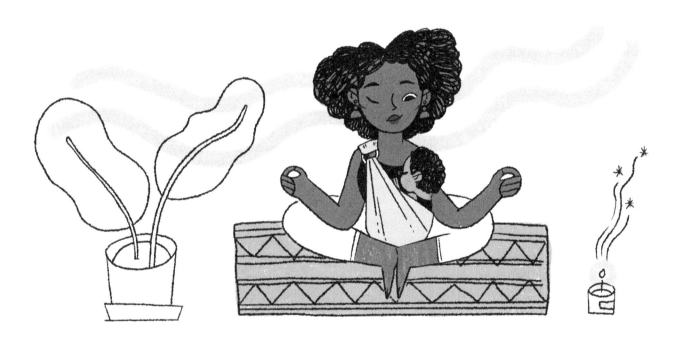

Meditation practice isn't about trying to throw ourselves away and become something better. It's about befriending who we are already.

- Pema Chödrön

DOI: 10.4324/9781003144021-12

# Mindfulness

How often do you find yourself zoning out right now? Do you feel super spacey, like it's really hard to focus on even the simplest of tasks? Being a new parent is really tough. Sleep deprivation, being overwhelmed, and being isolated initially only add to the difficulties. It is common to be easily distracted and have the attention span of a squirrel.

In general, there are many distractions that keep us from being focused on the present. We are constantly barraged by social media and email notifications, and even times with friends are interrupted by unwanted distractions. Becoming a parent causes us to be even more distracted in our daily lives. Attending to your child's safety, attuning to their (never ending!) cues and needs, as well as preparing for the next task can all be quite challenging. It's hard to focus as a parent, sometimes. How many times do you find yourself wondering why you walked into a room? Or how many times have you found yourself taking over an hour to finally finish a meal because you keep getting pulled away?

How often are you distracted by thinking about the constant tasks that are required as part of being a new mom, i.e. "When do I need to feed her again?", "Is he whining because he is sleepy or needs another diaper change?", "When should I buy more baby food? Can I grab a brief nap while she's napping or what if she's not down long enough?" These are common thoughts that run through the heads of every new parent. And, if you're also struggling with self-defeating thoughts that are typical with pregnancy and postpartum mood changes, then your lack of focus can be even more pronounced!

*Sarah's brain is on overdrive. She feels like she is just going through the motions and just barely staying on top of taking care of her baby. She feels like she is in a "time-lapse" video, she is moving so quickly from one task to the next, she is not sure, honestly, when she last went to the bathroom or showered and even which boob she last nursed from. And her brain! Her brain is constantly going, whether she is blaming herself for something she did wrong, or worrying about something coming up – she can't turn it off. Yesterday she was "playing" with her baby for a bit, and realized the whole thirty minutes she had been worrying instead about going back to work. She felt so guilty she wasted that whole time with her daughter, and in general feels really disconnected from both her baby and her spouse.*

When experiencing all the mood changes that come with having a baby, it is common to have thoughts of distraction and thoughts which focus on the future or the past, such as: "It won't get easier until she sleeps through the night" or "Everything was better before I had a baby." While these thoughts may be highlighting the difficulty of your present situation and speaking your truth, they can also contribute to a sense of helplessness because it is not helping you address what is happening now.

To be mindful means to bring your awareness to the present. Even if the present is a place of discomfort it can be a place of acceptance, even momentary acceptance, of where you are. And wherever you are in that moment is the only thing that is real (the catastrophic future you are predicting does not exist, and as hard as it is to accept, the past you are grieving is no longer here). And, if the present is a place of connection, joy, and peace, well, then what a wonderful place to bring awareness to and to learn how to be fully engaged! And, if the present is a place of sadness or discomfort, then it is where you are right now and it will pass!

# So, why mindfulness?

You are going through a lot of mood and life changes right now, right? It's a lot to manage. The purpose of being mindful is to keep you fully engaged where you are and to slow down, learn how to ground yourself into the present, soothe yourself, and just be. Mindfulness is not a way of learning how to

---

**Did You Know?**

- Mindfulness means catching the moments of enjoyment: when you are feeling calm, loving the sound of your baby's laughter, enjoying a second of quiet to yourself.

- Mindfulness is also just noticing the tough moments: "I feel overwhelmed and unhappy right now."

- In other words, those tough moments are temporary and going to pass.

---

be happy at all times but to learn how to effectively feel your feelings. Mindfulness practices can be particularly helpful if you are struggling with anxiety, racing thoughts, worrying, or bipolar symptoms. Mindfulness practices can also help decrease inflammation (Rosenkranz et al., 2013), help us tune into the body, and help us be in the moment. Of course you have many things to be preoccupied with at this time and we appreciate that. So how can you help yourself be more present and more in the moment?

## How can I practice mindfulness?

It might feel like a joke to ask you to practice mindfulness when your mind is a hamster wheel or your life feels like a dumpster fire. Mindfulness is simply an act of awareness. So when you catch yourself not being in the moment, it is important to practice bringing yourself to the moment.

**Step 1:** The first step of awareness is in fact catching yourself when you are not present. This in itself can be so hard! How might you know you are not present? If your mind is racing, if you are doing a million things at once, feeling frantic, overwhelmed, or "out of your body", you might not be present. If you are stuck worrying about the past or focused on something terrible happening in the future, you are likely not present.

**Step 2:** Once you "catch" yourself, you can begin to pay attention to your different senses to help bring you back to the present. For example, if you are with your baby, look carefully at the folds in her skin, the different colors within her eyes, the shape of her ear. Pay attention to the smells around you: the smell of her hair, her lotion, her clothes. Listen to the noises around you; your baby's gurgle, a cry, a burp. Pay attention to the feel of things near you; the roughness of a towel, the softness of your baby's skin. Added bonus: all of these things aid in promoting secure attachment which we have talked about before as well!

The act of paying attention to your senses can help bring you back into the moment. It allows you to be present versus missing moments around you and this can help when you are struggling with racing thoughts of an awful future or depressive thoughts of being stuck in the past. "But what if I'm not happy in the present right now?" you ask. That is OK! Not only is it ok but the whole purpose of this workbook is to remind you that it is common to feel off right now. Being present means allowing yourself to feel your feelings, whatever they are, in the moment.

## Activity

Close your eyes for 20 seconds when your baby is quiet or asleep. As your eyes are closed, listen to the sounds around you. What do you hear? Smell the smells around you. What are you experiencing? Touch the area around you. What do you feel?

Try and practice this three times a day and mark how you feel. Also, notice how mindfulness feels for you.

| Stress Level Before (0–10) | Day of Practice | Time of Day | Stress Level After (0–10) |
|---|---|---|---|
| | | | |
| | | | |
| | | | |
| | | | |
| | | | |

## Five Senses

Another mindfulness practice we like is called "the five senses".

1. Look around you and name five things you can see. Describe them in detail to yourself, paying attention to the small aspects of the item such as color, texture, shape, memory the item elicits, etc. Now take a deep, cleansing breath.

2. Now, name and feel four things you can touch, doing the same as above, to take time in describing the feel of each object. Now take a deep cleansing breath.

3. Now, slow down, listen and name three things you can currently hear. Take another deep cleansing breath.

4. Name two things you can smell. (Sometimes you have to "cheat" on this one and find something near you to smell such as clothes or food). Take another deep breath.

5. Now name one thing you can taste, and finish this practice with a breath.

How are you feeling? This practice helps you slow down and is particularly helpful when panicking, experiencing racing or obsessive thoughts, or needing to feel grounded in the present.

Allow yourself to be present, aware, and mindful. Remember, it is a practice to be mindful. Practice this exercise several times a day. This is a brief "microbreak" that you can learn to practice even as a busy new parent. We know you are busy, and if you don't want to use this space to write it down, it's fine. As always, use this workbook in a way that is easiest for you!

| Stress Level Before (0–10) | Day of Practice | Time of Day | Stress Level After (0–10) |
|---|---|---|---|
| | | | |
| | | | |
| | | | |
| | | | |
| | | | |

## MEDITATION

*OHMMMMMMM ....*

Meditation does not just have to be in a temple retreat at the top of a mountain. As a new parent, we know you do not have time for that (although the idea of running away to a mountaintop may be tempting)!

In this section, we want to tell you about the incredible things your brain is doing, and then help you learn to calm it down.

During your pregnancy and postpartum period, your brain is undergoing one of the most dramatic changes it will ever experience. You are experiencing hormonal fluctuations throughout each trimester while you are pregnant. Also, the birth of your baby, and even attachment and breastfeeding create new circuits of your brain which are being primed, enabling you to bond and respond to your baby's cues, develop empathy, etc. (Barba-Müller, Craddock, Carmona, & Hoekzema, 2019). It truly is an incredible time.

Researchers are really just beginning to learn about the brain's changes during motherhood as well as during times of sustained stress and trauma. For example, we are learning that when a person has experienced a traumatic event (e.g. a traumatic birth experience, baby in the NICU, postpartum complications, etc.) or chronic stress (e.g. perinatal anxiety or depression), there actually can be structural changes to the brain (van der Kolk, 2015).

### Did You Know?

- The prefrontal cortex, which is the part of the brain responsible for the higher-level executive functioning, logic, reasoning, and impulse control, **can shrink**.

- The hippocampus, the part of the brain responsible for memory storage, learning, and our self-awareness **can also grow smaller** which means it can become more difficult for us to form memories, hold awareness of ourselves, and learn valuable skills (ever feel like you are in Groundhog Day experiencing the same day over and over?).

- The amygdala, which is responsible for the fight/flight/freeze response, **can actually thicken and grow,** which means that we can have an enhanced state of awareness of our surroundings. This hyper awareness often brings feelings of anxiety and/or obsessive thoughts.

## The Good News

So, we know we just hit you with some nerdy information about how your brain can change with stress. But here's the good news: you can do something about it, and the brain can heal and recover!

The amazing news is that research shows that reparative changes to the brain can occur when we practice regular meditation or other calming practices (Holzel et al., 2011; Lazar et al., 2005). With meditation, the gray matter density increases in the Hippocampus, decreases in the Amygdala, and thickens in the Prefrontal Cortex, impacting the changes mentioned above. This is called *post-traumatic growth* and is a remarkable process. To summarize, all the negative brain changes we discussed above can be healed with calming practices like meditation and breathing practices. This helps us quiet our racing minds, build improved attention spans, have better memories, and feel an internal sense of calm.

## How You Can Interweave Meditation As a New Mom

You might be thinking "what new mother has time for meditation?". We are not talking about going to a meditation retreat or having an hour-long quiet time. Even if you can incorporate only small moments of breathing practices or meditation into your day, it can really help with these brain changes. Even five-minute meditation practices a few times a week can be particularly beneficial if you are experiencing mood changes during your pregnancy or after having a baby.

Meditation and breathing techniques can be helpful tools to help manage symptoms that occur with stress and trauma, particularly in conjunction with therapy or other treatments. And, let's face it, every new parent can use some little breaks and some breathing space!

*Talia was so exhausted after spending what seemed like hours getting her son down for a nap (although it was really just twenty-five minutes). She was agitated and frustrated and so emotionally spent. Once he was down, she plopped herself on the couch and stared blankly at the wall. She really didn't want to do anything while her son napped except zone out on a TV show. But she had promised herself she would try to incorporate some meditation in her day. So, she found a ten-minute meditation to help relieve stress. She felt a little better after that, and less on edge. Plus, she was proud of herself for taking some time just for her. Talia turned on her show after that and enjoyed the time to herself while her son napped. She noticed her mood was lighter when he awoke and was a little more calm.*

## Activity

Meditation can be particularly helpful during times of transition. Even a five-minute meditation exercise a few times a week can be helpful (we like several free meditation apps and have shared some options under the Resources chapter):

- when your baby is napping
- before your start into the next item on your "to-do" list
- before going to bed to quiet your mind
- sitting in the car before coming back inside while your baby is asleep in the car seat, etc.
- after feeding your baby at night if you are having difficulty falling back asleep

Choose one of your favorite meditation apps and write it here. Download it on to your phone now so that when you need it in the middle of the night to help you fall back to sleep, you already have it ready to go. We've given you some suggestions in our Resources chapter.

## Body Scan

Most people, when learning how to meditate, find they prefer to have someone guide them through it, which is why we recommend you try an app or guided video first. If you would like to practice a brief meditation exercise on your own, a body scan can be a good place to start. If you find you have difficulty tolerating this (racing mind, uncomfortable body sensations, etc.) this is not uncommon and we would encourage you to practice with a guided meditation. In fact, many women who have experienced trauma have difficulty tuning into their bodies at times. So if this is your experience, you are not alone and we recommend specifically searching for trauma informed body scans or trying modifications that work for you, like keeping your eyes open or sitting upright rather than lying down.

After reading the instructions, try to find a quiet space in your house if possible, such as while the baby is napping. You can have calming music on if you prefer.

1. Sit in a comfortable position or lie down with your body comfortably supported.
2. First, notice and tune into your breaths. No need to force your breathing to be anything other than what it is. Just notice the rhythm of your chest and belly rising and falling.
3. With time, shift your attention to the top of your head, and notice any sensations you have there. The purpose of today's body scan is truly just to scan, as if you had a magnifying glass. We are scanning and noticing, not trying to change or force.
4. Now, shift your attention to your face, jaw, and neck. Notice what you're feeling, and if you're holding any tension.
5. Bring awareness now to your shoulders and chest, paying attention to any tightness, tensions, or other sensations. Pause here, noticing again your breathing.
6. Now notice your arms from your shoulders down to your hands, maybe even wiggling your fingers.
7. Bring your attention back to your torso, stomach and back. This may be difficult, or not, given that this is a place where you are holding, or have held, your baby, and may be still recovering. Just notice, as you shift attention back to your breath.
8. Notice now your legs, paying attention all the way down to your feet, perhaps wiggling your toes.

9. As we close out today's practice, let's return your focus back to your breath, perhaps taking one deep cleansing breath. Please thank yourself for the practice you did today, no matter how successful you felt.

**How do you feel in your body? Do you feel more physically relaxed? How do you feel emotionally after that practice?**

_____

_____

**When setting a goal for meditation, how often would you like to try to practice bringing in some brief meditation into your week?**

_____

_____

## BREATHING RETRAINING

Do you ever find yourself getting panicky, feeling short of breath, or excessively yawning?

First, let's go over the nerdy stuff.

Mindful breathing can also be a helpful skill for regulating emotion, particularly if you are struggling with anxiety, intrusive thoughts, irritability, rage, bipolar symptoms, or if you have experienced trauma. Faulty or inefficient breathing patterns can make you more susceptible to panic and anxiety (Meuret, Wilhelm, & Roth, 2003). Some people who experience panic tend to have patterns of subtle hyperventilation breathing (Hegel & Ferguson, 1997). That means that they are generally breathing a little faster than is optimal and a flight or fight response can be more easily triggered.

### Did You Know?

- A person with chronic faulty breathing patterns can be subtly hyperventilating without their knowledge.
- It seems that their body has generally adjusted to their breathing pattern.
- Now it just takes a gasp, snore, or more rapid breathing to trigger the fight or flight response.
- People who have inefficient breathing patterns are more susceptible to panic attacks.

Learning how to breathe diaphragmatically can help. What that means is, instead of breathing superficially from the top of your chest, learning how to breathe from the deep part of your belly. Breathing diaphragmatically on a regular basis can reduce the susceptibility to panic attacks. We provided some references for diaphragmatic breathing in our Resources chapter.

# Activity

Place one hand on your chest and the other on your belly, if tolerable. As you breathe in and out, notice the rhythm of your breath and be mindful of allowing your belly to fill up with air like a balloon when you inhale, and deflate with exhalation. Try practicing this when:

- *frustrated* (You are stopped, stuck in traffic and your baby is crying in their car seat)
- *anxious* (You are having an intrusive thought and while telling yourself "this is anxiety, not real")
- *irritable* (You notice your irritability growing or when you are becoming angry)
- *overwhelmed* (You are feeling frustrated at your baby's cry)
- *sleepless* (You are in bed trying to fall asleep after feeding baby)

We recommend you practice for two minutes twice per day.

Added bonus: when you are in the midst of feeling stressed or anxious, slowing your breathing down can be calming enough to slow your thinking down and allow for more rational thinking.

## Other breathing options

**"Square breathing"** involves breathing in by a count of four seconds, holding for about four seconds, and breathing out for four seconds. Then pause for four seconds before resuming the pattern again. Because each count is by four, you are essentially forming a square with your breathing.

It is important that you're breathing by your counts and not by someone else's timing, as some people find it hard to tolerate this breathing exercise and may find it too slow if going at someone else's pace. People who like this breathing exercise and find that the counting is helpful may want to start with a "small square" by breathing in, holding the breath and exhaling for fewer seconds at a time and then building to a larger count. You can also hold a square pillow on your chest and trace the edges with your hands as you count.

**"Sip breathing"** involves taking two to three small "sips" of breath in and then slowly exhaling out in one long breath. This can often be more tolerable for those who are feeling panicky or still learning to be more comfortable in their bodies. This is especially useful for people with breathing issues (i.e. asthma) or people who have experienced trauma.

Find which breathing exercises you prefer; this is definitely not a one-size-fits-all, and it's important you do what works for you!

Hint: breathing exercises are brief and easy. If you do not have much time, a breathing exercise may be a doable one- to two-minute activity to incorporate throughout your day.

## Activity

**1. Set two times per day to practice the diaphragmatic breathing retraining for about two minutes. Record your practices, if you prefer.**

Date                  Difficulty Practicing (rate on scale 0–10)            # minutes practiced

_____

_____

_____

_____

Notice if, with time, it becomes easier to practice. If you prefer, rather than laying down, practice breathing retraining sitting up.

Or:

**2. When you notice you are feeling physically stressed or anxious or are flooded with anxious thoughts practice square or sip breathing:**

Date                  Difficulty Practicing (rate on scale 0–10)            # minutes practiced

_____

_____

_____

_____

## RELAXATION PRACTICES

You know how when you're stressed out, and someone tells you to "calm down", you kind of want to freak out? It's not helpful when someone tells you to "relax". And yet, when we're stressed, it can be really helpful to help *ourselves* learn to calm and self-soothe.

When worried, anxious, or angry, it is difficult to think clearly and rationally. Imagine your brain is filled with little ping pong balls (just go with it). When you become more agitated, they move more and more quickly, bouncing into each other and causing quite a bit of chaos. It is difficult to think rationally when your brain is so stimulated by all of the balls bouncing into each other, making all the noise and distraction. However, if the balls can slow down or even deflate, it is like your brain has just taken a deep breath and you can now pay attention to your thoughts and your body again. This is essentially what is happening when we are in "emotionally reactive mode" and not thinking rationally. We might be in fight/flight/freeze mode, experiencing catastrophic and anxious thoughts. We are physically activated. By learning how to calm the body, we can learn to activate our parasympathetic nervous system, which is soothing and enables us to access more rational thoughts.

Helping your body to relax helps you feel more rational and logical. Relaxation exercises are not meant to put you to sleep (though they can!). They are just meant to help you feel more relaxed.

**Progressive Muscle Relaxation** (PMR) is one type of relaxation exercise and is often helpful in relaxing the body. We think it can be helpful to learn the basic concept behind PMR which is learning how to allow your muscles to relax.

1. For this exercise and explanation, let's start with noticing the top of your head, eyes and forehead, tensing the muscles for a count of five, and then relaxing all of the muscles simultaneously as you breathe out slowly. The goal is to aim for as deep of relaxation as possible, which will be different for each person. There is no "perfect" to achieve here. Sit with noticing this part of the body and your breath for about ten to fifteen seconds before you move to the next muscle group. This is not an exercise to rush.

2. Now pay attention to the muscles around your cheeks and jaw. Tense these for the same count of five, and relax them as you breathe out. Sit and notice your body for ten to fifteen seconds as well and do so with each muscle group from here onward.

3. Similarly, notice the muscles of your neck. Strain and tense these for a count of five, and relax them as you breathe out.

4. Now move to your shoulders and tighten these muscles for the same count, relaxing them as you breathe out slowly.

5. Let's now move to your arms, and tighten these muscles, releasing them as you breathe out.

6. Now let's notice your hands and fingers tightening and relaxing as you exhale.

7. Moving to your chest, notice the inhale and any tension, and any release as you exhale.

8. Noticing your abdomen contract, release any tension as you breathe out slowly.

9. Now let's move to your back. Notice any tightness and allow all muscles to become as relaxed as possible as you exhale.

10. Turning your focus to our pelvic floor and bottom (notice this may be triggering given what you've just experienced with birth and you can skip this section if so), breathe out through these muscles as well.

11. Pay attention now to your thighs, tightening them for the count of 5, and then releasing them with an exhale out.

12. As you shift your attention down your legs, tighten your knees and shins, relaxing the muscles as you breathe out.

13. And finally, tighten your feet and toe muscles, and release them with a slow deep breath out, perhaps wiggling your toes as a final thank you to yourself for a great practice.

Notice how this is similar to the body scan exercise you learned earlier in the chapter, with the added element of tightening and relaxing the muscles. Which one do you prefer?

For more PMR practice, we recommend that you look up some online videos or download some relaxation apps. We have several apps that we use in our Resources chapter.

## Important Takeaways

- Mindfulness allows us to be present in the now and can help us feel calmer and more in control.

- Meditation can reverse the changes to the brain caused by trauma and stress, and improve overall brain functioning resulting in a physical and mental calmness.

- Whether you are practicing diaphragmatic breathing retraining, square breathing, or sip breathing, breathing practices can help rewire the brain and calm the body and mind.

- Relaxation practices help us activate the parasympathetic nervous system, enabling us to be more calm, logical, and rational.

- All of these activities can be done in just brief moments and can be easily interwoven into a busy parent's life!

# Part III

# Additional Factors – Aspects of Your Life That Can Impact Your Mood

# CHAPTER 11

# EMBRACING MORE OF YOU

## *CULTURE, IDENTITY, AND MENTAL HEALTH*

**Bethany Warren, LCSW, PMH-C**
**Beth Creager Berger, Ph.D.**

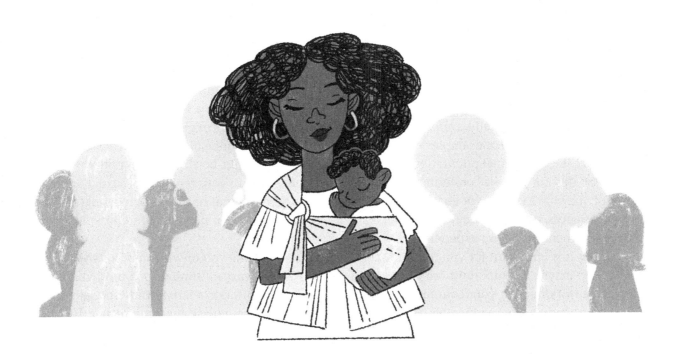

When I witness the resilience of women all over the world, rising above the most difficult situations, I am reminded that I can never give up.

- Zawadi Nyong'o

DOI: 10.4324/9781003144021-14

How does your identity and background impact your mental health? How have your life experiences shaped the way you are now responding to all the mood changes you are feeling now as a new parent?

As cisgender, White, straight, able-bodied women, we understand that we benefit from the privilege of this intersection of our identities. For example, when we see representations of motherhood in the media, they often look just like us. So, we want to inhabit this space with a place of humility and curiosity and want to be respectful of our language. Having worked with clients from diverse backgrounds in our careers, what we observe is that judgment from others, multigenerational trauma, and discrimination have an impact on mental wellbeing. Experiencing microaggressions or discrimination based on one's cultural identity has a compounding effect on what someone is already going through.

Our lived experiences are different based on the intersection of our various identities such as race, ethnicity, nationality, class, gender, sex, disability, religious identity, and size. Professor Kimberlé Crenshaw coined the term "intersectionality" in 1989 to explore how individual characteristics like those above intersect and overlap with one another and are not mutually exclusive (Crenshaw,1989). This theory highlighted systemic issues like inequality and discrimination, particularly with those faced by Black women.

We understand that people's experiences are significantly shaped by their full identities. For example, a Black, able-bodied, pregnant, straight, cisgender mother will have quite a different experience than that of a disabled, White, gay, pregnant mother. And, these lived experiences can have quite a significant impact on our mental health and access to care.

## Accessibility to Care

Perhaps you are already struggling with depressive symptoms and are finding it difficult to reach out to anyone in your community. Are there barriers to seeking help such as a lack of providers who are trained in providing culturally competent care in your area? This is where exploring intersectionality of your identity is helpful. For example, are you concerned that you might be discriminated against based on your size, race, or sexual orientation? Are you concerned you might be able to find a provider that has accessibility for your size or disability, but may not be affirming to your religious or sexual orientation? You may have mistrust or guardedness about the medical or mental health system based on your own experiences, or generational history. It can be really complicated for people to find providers that understand them. Have you experienced this?

Perhaps it is important for you to find other parents who look like you or who are from your community. Or, maybe it's important for you to work with providers who are similar to you or who have experience working with your community. Inclusivity and representation matters and especially now if you are already feeling vulnerable and struggling. Have you experienced anything related to your identity, culture, or sense of belonging that has had an impact on your mental health?

## What Is Culture?

Culture is essentially the way of life of a group of people. It can include our systems, attitudes, and feelings, and can include how we view ourselves, and our values. Culture can be our racial identity, our spiritual and religious beliefs, nationality, the groups we belong to, and even our professional way of life, such as belonging to military culture. Our cultural identity in addition to our other identities can be an important part of our sense of belonging. Not every part of our identity defines us, or is central to our social connections to others. Though for many, our connection to our cultural identity can be a way for us to feel bonded. Alternatively, there can also be distressing experiences around cultural identities. Have you ever had to downplay your identity in order to feel safe? Have you ever felt like your cultural identity was not respected by others? Let's explore more about how culture can interweave with parenthood.

## Activity

**List the various identities that you identify with.** (Examples might include race, ethnicity, nationality, class, gender, sex, sexual orientation, military affiliation, disability, marital status, religious identity, and body size.)

_____

_____

_____

_____

_____

_____

_____

**How have your various identities positively impacted you as a parent?** (For example: I am able bodied and had a fairly uncomplicated pregnancy; my culture was very mother-centric and my immediate community has supported me throughout my pregnancy and early recovery.)

_____

_____

_____

_____

_____

_____

## Belonging

Do you remember when you were younger and how you were super focused on anything that might set you apart from anyone else? From what you wore, to what you brought for lunch, there was often an intense pressure to fit in.

As we were writing this section, we were laughing reminiscing about all the shenanigans we pulled in order to fit in when we were younger. And the funny thing is, this pressure never goes away, the details just change as we become adults.

The need to belong is an innate desire, right? From an early age we see children and adolescents trying to find a place of belonging among their peers as they struggle against peer pressure. As an adult, the need to belong does not subside but takes on different forms. There are different groups where we find our belonging: the married group, the friends group, a mom's club, a religious social group, etc. And the peer pressure continues throughout our lives with questions such as: "When are you going to get married?", "When are you going to have children?", and the list goes on.

Parenthood can sometimes be fraught with inherent competitiveness, and questions from others are often judgmental and can be perceived as a judgment of your parenting skills or your abilities or worth as a mother (particularly when you are struggling with your own internal negative narrative). Questions such as: "Are you breastfeeding?", "Are you co-sleeping?", "Did you sign up to volunteer for your kid's class?", or "Are you giving your child organic food?" can make parents feel guilty and pressured.

**And, what if you belong to a group that is underrepresented with services or discriminated against?**

For new parents, there is incredible pressure from Day One. The pressure to fit in is intensified today with social media and a hyper-awareness on the "right" way to parent. Being a new mom can already breed feelings of not being good enough. To add to that, you may also experience stigma or discrimination from others due to your identity. As a new mom who identifies in a group that is stigmatized, how have you experienced feeling judged?

_____

_____

_____

Parents who face judgment or microaggressions are more at risk for perinatal mood symptoms given additional stressors and less available competent professional support. For instance, Black and Latina women are more likely to have Perinatal Mood and Anxiety disorders, and yet are less likely to be screened or treated for them (Kozhimannil et al., 2011). A study with transgender parents found that loneliness was a pervasive theme through each part of achieving gestational parenthood. (Ellis, Wojnar & Pettinato, 2014). Additional examples may include single mothers, other women of color, parents who conceived through surrogacy, parents who went through IVF, parents in same-sex relationships, parents of a child with a disability, older mothers, teenage moms, parents who are first generation in their country, etc. It would make sense that these parents are more at risk for perinatal mood symptoms.

---

### Did You Know?

- Women of color are at higher risk for PMADs than White women, with numerous studies showing that African-American, Latina, Indigenous, Pacific Islander and immigrant women are at greater risk than White women (Blustain, 2019; Lara-Cinisomo, Wisner, Burns, & Chaves-Gnecco, 2014).

- Native American women have consistently high prevalence rates of PMADs (Ko, Rockhill, Tong, Morrow, & Farr, 2017).

- One-third of Latina teenagers viewed their childbirth as traumatic and 50% of them had symptoms of trauma afterwards (Anderson, 2010).

- Depression is more common in single mothers than married mothers (Brown & Moran, 1997).

- PMADs are more common in lesbian mothers than heterosexual mothers (Ross, Steele, Goldfinger, & Strike, 2007).

---

_Julie is a White, lesbian mother, married to a Black woman. She gave birth to one child and they adopted another. Both children are Black. The stigmas and boneheaded questions Julie, her wife, and their children face can be exhausting at times. Exhausting on top of already being mama-exhausted. "Which one of you is the Dad?", "Are you the nanny?", "Which one is yours?" As a White woman, Julie describes having to constantly "come out of the closet" as gay or as having a biracial family because it may not be immediately obvious to people. When she is by herself, people make assumptions based on her race and socioeconomic status. Julie becomes exhausted having to constantly educate strangers on her family and how their questions are sometimes ignorant or rude. She describes that having to explain herself to others all the time is one more stressor on top of being a new mom. Julie recognizes her privilege as a White woman, but feels guilty at times, because despite her own experiences, her wife experiences outward discrimination much more frequently than she does._

## Activity

**What are some stigmas you think may exist as a result of your various identities or your cultural background?** (Stigmas might include: not being understood, being hated or judged, being cut off from family, being underrepresented in the media, etc.)

_____
_____
_____
_____
_____
_____
_____

**Have you ever been misunderstood, discriminated against, physically or verbally harmed because of any aspect of your culture or identity?** (Adapted from Nickerson, 2017.) If so, what happened?

_____
_____
_____
_____
_____
_____
_____

Every mom knows what it's like to feel judged. Women from cultures that historically and currently are targets of prejudice may feel constantly judged or under attack.

**Have you ever felt judged as a parent?** Examples might include your choice of co-sleeping, feeding method, attachment parenting, being a working parent, being a stay-at-home parent, having a babysitter for your child, or having your child in daycare)

_____
_____
_____
_____
_____
_____

_Nia was a newly single mom of two girls. She has tried really hard since her divorce to remain active in her children's lives. She coached her older daughter's softball team, was the classroom mom, and, after work, made sure to have nightly dinners together with her girls. Still she worried about others' judgments of her as a single mom. Recently, her baby rolled off the changing table. The pediatrician reassured her the baby was completely fine and would just have a bad bruise for a while. Although Nia was really concerned about her daughter she was also concerned that other parents would blame the incident on her for not being as attentive to her children because she is a single parent._

In the face of judgment from others coupled with the emotions you might be struggling with, it is important to remind yourself of the things you are doing well! You are a competent and loving parent.

**Name one thing that you are proud of as a parent.** Ideas might include how you are doing your best with feeding your child, you are proud of your bond with your baby, you love singing to your baby at night, etc.

_____

_____

_____

### How does our cultural identity impact our views on mental health?

We take the cue about a lot of our core values and what we hold dear to us based on those around us, and how we were raised. Our environment really shapes us. And with regard to mental health, we may have received messages around mental wellness. Perhaps you were raised around people who talk openly about feelings and emotions, and you saw emotional expression modeled. Maybe you even saw people going to therapy or taking medication when they struggled with mental illness. Or, on the other hand, perhaps mental illness was stigmatized in your community or family, and you were raised not to talk openly about feelings. Perhaps emotions were dealt with privately, or only in the home or religious community. As a result, you may be struggling now even more so with your heightened emotions if you feel like it is unacceptable to seek out help or tell others that you are not doing well.

_Mariana is a first generation Mexican American and ever since she had her baby, she is so sad. At the deepest part of her, she suspects there is something really wrong because she cries all the time, and it feels like the whole world is colored gray. She moves so slowly through all the motions of caring for her baby, and just can't find the joy in anything anymore. But when she tried to tell her mom and aunties how she was feeling, even though she knows they love her so much, it didn't go well. Mariana left the conversation feeling ashamed, like somehow she must be broken because her mom and aunties made it seem like motherhood is so great and she should feel lucky. No one seemed to understand why she is sad, and when she said she wanted to go on medication, they begged her not to. It feels like such a hard choice, like she's choosing between her family or her doctor's advice._

# Activity

We've just discussed some ways that your culture, or various aspects of your identity might impact your experience as a mother. **As you have been reading this book and learning about your experience and mood symptoms, can you think about how your culture and intersecting identities might impact how you are experiencing your mental health?**

_____

_____

_____

**What messages did you learn about mental illness as you were growing up?**

_____

_____

_____

**What are the messages around mental health treatment in your community?**

_____

_____

_____

**What is the availability of mental health treatment in your community?**

_____

_____

_____

_____

**Do you have any friends or family who have modeled that it is ok to get help for their mental health concerns?**

_____

_____

_____

_____

_____

## Other Considerations:

- What else is impacting your community right now?

- It can be important to consider what other traumatic events and daily stressors might be impacting your community that might also have an impact on your mental health.

- For example Latina immigrants were found to have four times the rates of PTSD than that of their White counterparts (Cleaveland & Frankenfeld, 2019).

## Finding Your Community

Parenting can be really isolating and hard, right? There's a reason why you probably keep hearing the phrase "it takes a village". One of the reasons for identifying at risk groups for developing Perinatal Mood and Anxiety mood symptoms is to pay attention to those who may need additional support. As we have talked about throughout this book, building a sense of community helps lessen the impact of mental illness and helps build a sense of belonging. This is particularly important in women who feel especially underrepresented with healthcare services or who feel unheard. Stigma, rejection or criticism from family and friends, bias, and a lack of services can impact this feeling of a lack of belonging as well. We all need a sense of belonging, and it is even more important to "find your community" and feel a sense of safety during motherhood. Finding support groups, play groups, and continuing to build your "village" will help you feel a sense of community and validation.

Having true support is so important, isn't it? Research shows us that positive social support and connectivity is a powerful protection against becoming overwhelmed by trauma and stress (Charuvastra & Cloitra, 2008). Because trauma often impacts our view of our world and our place in our world (with common negative thoughts, such as "I'm alone", "I'm defective"), positive support can help protect and rebuild these connections to our community. Secure connections with others help us build resiliency and allow us to feel less alone.

---

### Did You Know?

- Connections with others can help us:
  - build internal resiliency
  - connect with tangible resources
  - eliminate a sense of being an outside "other" (Landau & Saul, 2004; Chemtob, 2002; Seaburn, Landau-Stanton, & Horwitz, 1995).
- Connectivity to others can also help protect against mental illness.
- The number one predictor of those with PTSD that recover well are those who have support systems (Solomon, 1990).

---

Connection with social support is a tremendous buffer and this is shown across the globe. Meaningful and safe connections to others are fundamental foundations to our mental wellbeing. As new mothers, this is particularly crucial (and ironic that many mothers have an internalized belief that they must do this on their own and are showing weakness if they ask for help). Many cultures have traditions of surrounding new parents with support in the early postpartum recovery period. In China, for example, the "sitting the month" period entails the woman staying indoors with the baby to focus on bonding and nursing while others cook for her and tend to her needs. Even though multigenerational homes are no longer always the norm, this continues to be a mainstream practice. Similarly, in India, a confinement period around 40 days is often practiced where the new mother is fed, nurtured and supported while she focuses on healing and tending to the baby.

## Activity

**Does your community have a tradition or ritual of surrounding new parents with support? If so, what is this tradition?**

_____
_____
_____
_____

**Learning how important connection is to mental wellbeing and resilience, how might you build on your community?** (Ideas might be finding in-person support groups, online chat groups, social media groups, connections through your religious community or community center, play groups, etc. We encourage you, if you haven't found a good fit yet, to keep trying. It can be challenging to find a group where you feel completely comfortable as a new parent).

_____
_____
_____
_____
_____

**Do you have any questions or concerns about differences or similarities with any of your providers' (i.e. therapist, birth worker, lactation consultant) culture/identities that might impact your comfort and safety when working with them?** (Ideas might be asking your provider about their experience working with clients of color, antiracism or cultural competency trainings they have taken, etc.)

_____
_____
_____
_____
_____
_____
_____

**As a new parent, do you have any role models or support systems within your culture and your identities? What strengths do you admire in them that you would like to grow in yourself?**

_____
_____
_____

## Important Takeaways

- Parents from historically and current stigmatized, judged, and/or oppressed groups are more at risk for postpartum mood changes.
- Being stigmatized and having perceived judgment can even further affect your mood.
- The need to belong is innate and so crucial as parents.
- Finding community can help with a sense of belonging and support.

# CHAPTER 12

## HOW'S YOUR PARTNER DOING?

### *(YES, THEY CAN STRUGGLE TOO!)*

Bethany Warren, LCSW, PMH-C
Beth Creager Berger, Ph.D.

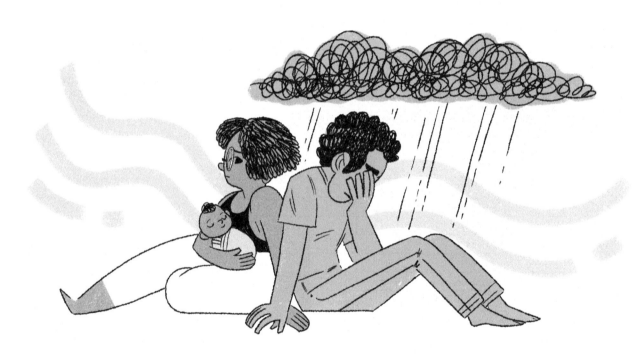

It's not that misery loves company, it's that company is the antidote to misery.

- Dr. Kristin Neff

DOI: 10.4324/9781003144021-15

Everyone always thinks it's the partner's job to support mom after having a baby. But here's the thing. They just became a parent and they need support too. Whether you are the non-birth partner, or you're the one who gave birth to your baby and you're worried about how your partner is faring in all of this, please keep reading. You may even want to work through this chapter together! As you have learned throughout this book, partners can also take an emotional hit throughout pregnancy (and especially during the postpartum phase as they too are adjusting to parenthood) and yet are often overlooked.

Partners can themselves experience an actual Perinatal Mood and Anxiety Disorder, and upwards of one in ten men will have a legitimate diagnosable PMAD (Paulson & Bazemore, 2010)! We have also seen that far too many spouses and partners will have a rough time adjusting to being a new parent. The common denominator, whether what they are experiencing is at a diagnosable level or not, is that most people don't ask dads and partners how they are doing.

## Did You Know?

- One in ten dads can develop a Perinatal Mood and Anxiety Disorder (Paulson & Bazemore, 2010).
- Lesbian mothers have a higher incidence of PMADs than heterosexual mothers (Ross, Steele, Goldfinger, & Strike, 2007).

In fact, in our experience, we are finding that often, even professionals, don't think to check on anyone but the birth parent. Adoptive parents and partners often seem to be left out of the conversation around mental health. Many obstetricians, pediatricians, and even friends don't ask how non-biological parents are doing (so you can assume then that partners certainly aren't officially being screened using any mood/symptoms screening scales). If you actually ARE a provider or friend who asks about the wellbeing of partners, then we dig your style.

## The Pressure on Partners:

If you have been overlooked, keep on reading, you are in the right place. Your life has just been turned upside down and we get it, it's a lot to adjust to. You too are also sleep-deprived, overwhelmed, anxious and stressed, feeling like you're faking it, and maybe even grieving your prior life that was flexible, fun and carefree. AND a lot of your family and friends are likely looking to you now, to support your partner when secretly you may be freaking out and wondering who is going to support YOU.

We don't do a good job of supporting dads and partners in our society, unfortunately, and we're sorry that that's the case. **Both of you** need a lot of support right now, and your sole support should not be just coming from each other. Each of the chapters involving self-care, accessing/building support networks and asking for help apply to you too. You also are adjusting to becoming a parent, and as such, you need your own team of support and your own practice of taking care of yourself in order to sustain this pace. Your roles have also changed, and the way you are interacting with your partner may feel vastly different. You may feel disconnected physically and emotionally, now, and that may feel scary.

## Activity:

If this is the first chapter you are reading as the non-birth partner, welcome! Again, most of this workbook can apply to you too, (even though this chapter is all about you). We recommend that you go now to Chapter 1 to familiarize yourself with the book and see what other chapters may interest you, such as the chapter on self-care, role changes and relationships, and how to manage your thoughts.

In addition, we want to ask, how are YOU doing? Partners can also get depression, anxiety, trauma symptoms, and even more serious symptoms such as bipolar and psychotic mood changes when having a baby sometimes. And just like birthing, adoptive, or gestational moms, partners also deserve support so these mood changes can be normalized and addressed.

**So, what are you feeling right now?** Please put a checkmark next to anything you are experiencing currently, or over the past 2 weeks.

**Symptom checklist:**

Racing thoughts _____ Worrying/anxiety _____ Panic attacks_____ Fears _____

Difficulty concentrating _____ Change in appetite _____ Loss of interest in activities _____

Irritability _____ Anger_____ Depression _____ Sadness _____ Hopelessness _____

Sleep problems _____ Loss of energy_____ Weight changes _____ Memory changes _____

Grief/loss _____ Tearfulness _____ Lack of motivation _____ Low self-esteem _____

Easily frustrated _____ Hyperactivity _____ Euphoria _____ Impulsivity _____

Relationship issues _____ Sexual issues _____ Mood swings _____ Feeling empty _____

Flashbacks _____ Nightmares _____ Disorientation _____ Confusion _____

*Seeing things others do not _____ *Self-harm _____ *Suicidal thoughts _____

*Hearing things others do not _____ *Feeling paranoid _____

*If you have checked any of the last two rows of symptoms, please seek outside help with a professional because it is important for you to have additional support right now. The Resources chapter has some good recommendations.*

**Body sensations:**

Fatigue _____ Body/muscle tension _____ Headaches _____

Stomachaches _____ Chest pain _____ Increased restlessness _____

**What was this experience like marking down the symptoms you are feeling?**

_____

_____

_____

**Were any of your symptoms above surprising to you?**

_____

_____

_____

**And what could you use right now (even if you don't know where you would get it yet)?**
Ideas might be: alone time, time with friends, more laughter, more time with your partner, validation you are still important to your partner, reassurance that what you're feeling is normal, professional mental health help, etc.

_____

_____

_____

_____

Are you surprised by what you wrote down? Or, perhaps you found it difficult to write anything down out of shame or embarrassment. Maybe you feel like you should still be the one still keeping it together for your family. Or maybe you're overwhelmed and don't know where to start. The story we tell ourselves can be powerful and often guides our actions, and perhaps you're feeling stuck or withdrawing. More help on addressing your thoughts can be found in Chapters 7 and 8.

*Darryl feels like a failure of a father and husband. Ever since they had their baby girl, he has felt so overwhelmed. Even though his wife says she's having a hard time, and he sees her crying and saying she's depressed, she still seems so capable of taking care of their daughter. But he just can't seem to do anything right. He's terrified of every little interaction with their baby; it feels like he can't soothe her when she's crying, and he secretly wonders if she doesn't even really like him. But he doesn't want to say anything because isn't he supposed to be the one that has it all together? All of their friends and family only ask about his wife and baby, and how they're doing. Everyone seems to assume he's fine and so he fakes that he is, when inside he wants to scream. He knows he's becoming more and more irritable, and more withdrawn from his wife and less engaged in taking care of their baby, but he doesn't know what to do.*

**How has having a baby impacted your relationship?**

In the chapter on role changes, we talked a lot about the strain that you are both under now as a couple, and how so many of your relationship dynamics have now changed. You may have previously felt quite capable of being a provider, "the strong one", or believed yourself to be fairly independent even in your relationship. It can be really difficult when key aspects of us are temporarily changed when having a baby! When we believed ourselves to be the "strong provider" previously, for example, and now we feel vulnerable and scared, it can be particularly nerve wracking to have to admit our fears to others or ask for help.

> **Did You Know?**
>
> • Remember, becoming a parent has an impact on your relationship.
>
> • This can be a hard time for most couples to navigate.
>
> • Upwards of 67% of couples report marital dissatisfaction after having a baby (Gottman & Gottman, 2007).
>
> • In other words, you're not alone!

Perhaps you feel overlooked in your relationship now. Or, maybe, you even feel jealous of your partner and baby's relationship and miss the closeness that you used to feel. Maybe you even wonder sometimes if you made the right choice in having children, or miss your old life. While these feelings aren't often discussed publicly, we hear them frequently in our offices. Having a baby changes things, and in particular, having a baby has a huge impact on the relationship.

This is now a good time to remind you that **you are not alone**. There is nothing wrong with you for feeling different or overwhelmed right now. You are a new parent and adjusting to this new role is hard! Having connections with others can be really useful. You may not feel ready to share how you are feeling with your partner yet, but it is important that you are able to express your struggles too.

**Who might you reach out to for support right now?** Ideas might be friends who are also parents, close family members or friends who are supportive and easy to talk to, etc.

_____

_____

**Do you ever wonder when you're going to "get her back"?**
Perhaps not only are you having a challenging time adjusting to parenthood, but you are also watching your partner struggling with her adjustment, and it seems she is having a rough time as well. And this might be scary wondering when you're going to "get her back" and not knowing exactly how to help her, much less you. (Insider tip: she's likely wondering when she is going to "get herself back" as well, so it can be really useful to talk to each other about this and your expectations).

_Anne feels ashamed to admit this so she hasn't told a soul, but she's jealous of their baby. She really misses their old life, back when it was just her and her wife, pre-baby. They were so free, and fun, and seemed to have a pretty good relationship, all things considered. And even though they desperately wanted a baby, and worked really hard to have him, now that he is here, it seems everything is different. Anne's wife loves being a mom and loves their son. She seems really into breastfeeding, wearing their baby, and seems really bonded with him. Even though Anne loves seeing this side of her wife, she secretly feels really sad and envious of the time she's lost with her. She feels like she got replaced, and wonders if they'll ever feel close again. And though she loves their son too, she wonders if she just doesn't love him like her wife does, and that makes her feel like an awful person. So she just stays quiet, and sad, and ashamed._

You are not alone. Many partners find support from other parents quite useful during this time for reassurance, validation, and tangible suggestions. At the end of the book in the Resources Chapter, we have resources for partners, too, such as online support groups, chat forums, and great articles to read. It can be liberating to hear from others who are experiencing the same thing that you are, particularly if you have been feeling isolated and alone.

**What is one thing you wish your partner knew about how you were feeling right now?**

_____

_____

**What would it be like to share this with her?** For example: "I'm afraid I'll burden her because she's already got too much going on", or "I'm just angry and resentful so I'm not sure it would go well", or "I've never really been that vulnerable with her before so it would be weird but might feel like a relief to get it off my chest".

_____

_____

_____

_____

If you do worry that telling your partner what you're feeling may burden her, we can reassure you that we often hear that from our mom clients themselves, worrying about telling their partners what _they_ are feeling. And yet, when they do, there is often relief in sharing in order to now move forward together.

It is said that families are like baby mobiles. We are all interconnected, and that what impacts one of us, impacts all of us (both good and bad). And while we may think that we are helping our partner by staying silent with our struggles, our partners often suspect we are struggling and they worry. Instead, we can draw strength from being interconnected as a couple. It can feel like a relief that you do not have to fight these struggles alone. You are a team, after all.

**And, what is one thing you wish you could hear from your partner that would provide some reassurance?**

_____

_____

**Notice that. What might you do with that?** (Examples include telling her your concerns, using skills learned from Chapter 9 to voice your needs directly, asking your partner for reassurance).

_____

_____

## Important Takeaways

- If you are experiencing any changes in your mood after having a baby, you are not alone! Up to one in ten partners will experience an actual Perinatal Mood and Anxiety Disorder (PMAD) themselves, and many more report difficulty adjusting to parenthood, sleep deprivation and relationship changes with their partners.

- Up to 67% of couples report marital dissatisfaction after having a baby, so if you are noticing changes in your relationship, it is common and something that you can address when you're ready.

- Whatever you are experiencing as a new parent, you are not alone, and it is not solely your responsibility to support your partner. You need support too!

# CHAPTER 13

# CRYING, LOW SEX DRIVE, IRRITABILITY AND MORE

## *HOW YOUR HORMONAL AND BIOLOGICAL CHANGES IMPACT YOUR EMOTIONS*

Bethany Warren, LCSW, PMH-C
Beth Creager Berger, Ph.D.

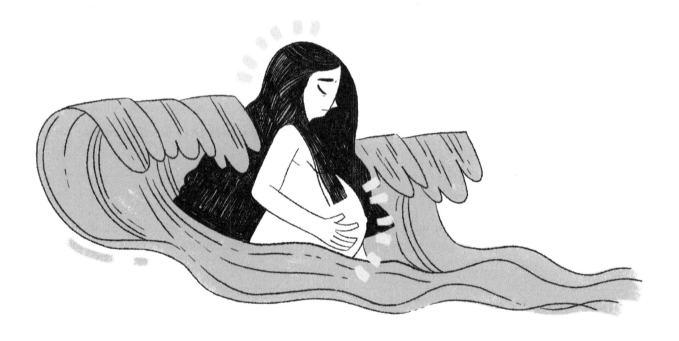

Normalize messy healing. It won't always be pleasant, it's rarely straightforward, and landing softly can be challenging. Your healing doesn't have to be a pretty picture of resilience.

- Alex Elle

DOI: 10.4324/9781003144021-16

## Hormonal and Biological Changes During Pregnancy

Don't you hate it when you're emotional and someone says to you "are you on your period?" This totally minimizes whatever you are feeling, right? Our emotions are completely valid, no matter what. And yet . . .

There is a strong link between hormones, mood, and physical symptoms. But our emotions are still totally valid! Our emotions can be exaggerated during this time, but they are real. When you are experiencing hormonal fluctuations (like PMS, pregnancy, the first year after having a baby, or menopause) your emotions are legitimate but it's like the volume gets turned up.

In Chapter 7, we helped you identify some of the underlying thoughts that may be impacting your mood. Negative thoughts and worry can cause physical symptoms associated with depression and anxiety (for example worrying can be associated with chest tightness),

In this chapter, we wanted to help you learn about some of the common biological and hormonal triggers to your current mood as well. Physical symptoms often trigger the negative thoughts associated with depression and anxiety (for example, feeling lightheaded might trigger thoughts of worrying something catastrophic is wrong with your physical health). Hormonal changes often manifest with significant physical symptoms. This helps explain why we often see mood changes during times of hormonal fluctuations.

### Did You Know?

- The most common times of onset of mood disorders for women are:
- during menses
- during and after pregnancy
- with the first menstruation post-pregnancy
- when weaning breastfeeding
- during menopause (Soares & Zitek, 2008).

The changes in hormones during pregnancy, particularly estrogen and progesterone, can directly affect mood. First, we will give you some helpful information to explain a few of the hormonal changes that occur during and after pregnancy that you might experience. Then, we will talk about some things that you can do to manage mood symptoms related to this.

### Estrogen and Progesterone

It's not you, it's your hormones. Ok, it's at least partly your hormones. Estrogen and Progesterone increase significantly during pregnancy which affect the level of neurotransmitters in the brain. These hormones then significantly decrease in the immediate postpartum period. Neurotransmitters affect and regulate mood. The rise and fall of estrogen and progesterone during pregnancy and after pregnancy can cause symptoms of depression and anxiety for some women. (Skalkidou, Hellgren, Comas, Sylvein, & Poromaa, 2012; Hall & Steiner, 2013). While hormones can be somewhat out of your control, this can be important information to have when you may have wondered "why has this happened to me?". Having knowledge can be empowering.

## Human Chorionic Gonadotropin (hCG) and Nausea

*Natalia wants to know the person who called it "morning sickness" so she can kick them in the shin. This nausea lasts all day long and sometimes even her heartburn wakes her up in the night. She barfs at the littlest smell, she's exhausted all the time, and just wants to lay on her couch and stare at the ceiling. Natalia is so resentful of the cute pregnant ladies with that adorable glow and those little adorable baby bumps. She feels huge and gross and doesn't want to go out in public. She feels angry all the time and so scared. Every time she gets nauseated, she can't help but wonder if there's something really wrong, and if she's going to lose the baby. There seems to be nothing anyone can say that will make her feel better, and she can't wait for this all to be over. She feels so ashamed of these feelings, though, and so sad she's missing out on the fun part of pregnancy.*

Did you experience nausea during your pregnancy? Nausea is really common during pregnancy, and can contribute to feelings of helplessness, exhaustion, powerlessness, overall depression, and anxiety.

hCG levels double every two days during the first ten weeks of pregnancy. It is possible that rising hCG levels are related to the nausea and vomiting that often occurs during pregnancy (Herrell, 2014). These are some common thoughts women experience when they are nauseous **(check any that you may have experienced)**:

- ☐ Will I ever get better?
- ☐ Will I be ok?
- ☐ Why me?
- ☐ Is there something really wrong with me? (or the baby)
- ☐ What if I throw up again?
- ☐ I'm so exhausted, how can I handle this?
- ☐ What if this keeps happening, how am I going to handle this for months and months?
- ☐ What if this is permanent?
- ☐ How can I go out? I might get sick in public.

And for many women, the physiological sensation of nausea can be distressing itself and triggering to anxiety and panic episodes. For women who experience ongoing nausea, this can lead to feelings of helplessness and hopelessness, which can then impact mood. Complications, such as hyperemesis (severe or prolonged vomiting), can be risk factors for mood symptoms during pregnancy as well. If you experienced (or are experiencing) this, it is important to think about how this may have impacted your current mood.

### Did You Know?

- The experience of nausea during pregnancy can be really traumatic for a lot of women.
- In fact, there is a significant association between the severity of nausea experienced, and a woman's risk of developing posttraumatic stress symptoms (Kjeldgaard et al., 2019).

**This roller coaster of hormones not only affects mood but also can affect libido as well. Let's explore how it can impact the emotional and physical connection with your partner**.

## Let's Talk About Sex . . .

Do you even want to? It's ok if your instinct was to skip this section entirely, in fact, many of our clients have a difficult time talking about sex both during and after their pregnancies. And it makes sense that talking about sex may be uncomfortable, particularly if you think there is something physically wrong with you. Let us reassure you, there is nothing wrong with you! There are huge changes that happen biologically, hormonally, emotionally, and physically during this time that often have an impact on libido (not to mention the impact on relationships, as we discussed in Chapter 9). You may feel as if your body has been hijacked and has changed. You may have even had a traumatic or difficult delivery, making sexual intimacy painful or uncomfortable. Or, you may have no desire to resume intimacy because you're exhausted, your body no longer feels like your own, and it feels like it now belongs to your baby. You may feel "all out of love", so to speak, and "over-touched."

You may have had an episiotomy or tearing, a cesarean section, or pelvic floor damage. You might still be recovering from significant body changes. What's happening hormonally and biologically also has a significant impact. It is common for the many changes after delivery to have a negative impact on sex drive (Hughes, 2008). And even more so if you're experiencing mood changes because mood symptoms can also have an impact on lowered libido.

It's ok if you aren't ready yet to resume sexual intimacy. Intimacy can take many forms, including physical touch and closeness, time spent together, sexual gestures, and intercourse. And it can be common for women after delivery to not only need time to recover (and this is variable for each woman), but for couples to need time to find ways to reconnect after baby. Listen to your body and what you need.

*Mei has zero interest in sex. In fact, at her postnatal visit when she got physical clearance to resume sexual intimacy, she was half hoping that her ObGyn would read her body language and tell her in front of her partner that she wasn't physically ready to have sex yet. Mei was really hoping her doctor wasn't going to give her the "green light". And it's not just that things have changed physically down there (though wow have things changed). Mei feels so over-touched and overstimulated after constantly being with and holding her baby all day, she has nothing left to give anyone else. And coupled with that is feeling so hypervigilant and anxious all the time; it would be virtually impossible to let her mind focus on her partner and allow herself to be in the moment. She feels guilty sometimes because she knows this is becoming "a thing" in her relationship, but part of her is too exhausted to be able to address it fully. So, instead, she's hoping her attempts at snuggling on the couch are ok. After all, that's the best she can do right now.*

Low sex drive during the postpartum period can be common. Keep checking in with yourself and your partner for ways to connect/reconnect during this time.

## Activity:

You may not be ready to resume sexual intercourse yet but there are other things that you can do to promote emotional and physical reconnection with your partner. Ideas can include **(check any that you feel comfortable with exploring):**

☐ Going for walks together

☐ Planning time alone

☐ Watching a favorite movie together

☐ Revisiting favorite memories together (i.e. looking through a photo album)

☐ After the baby goes to bed, spending some quality time talking together

☐ Holding hands

☐ Staying connected throughout the day

☐ Cuddling on the couch

☐ Kissing and/or hugging

☐ Massage or gentle touch

☐ Another idea for emotional and physical connection I have is:

## Hormonal Sensitivity, Difficult Periods, and Endometriosis

You know how we all have that girlfriend who is barely impacted by her period? And then, on the other hand, we know friends who are knocked down during their period, and severely impacted by their symptoms. Some women have a really difficult time during the week leading up to their periods with increased irritability, moodiness, tearfulness, and even rage. Other women do not experience this at all. There seems to be a range of experiences, right? We know that some women are more sensitive to hormonal changes in their body than other women. You may tend to be more emotionally sensitive during times of hormonal shifts such as menses, pregnancy, postpartum and perimenopause. Research actually shows that some women tend to have more of a hormonal sensitivity than other women during these different times throughout their lifespan (Pope, Oinonen, Mazmanian & Stone, 2017).

PMDD, Premenstrual Mood Dysphoric Disorder, for example, is similar to PMS (Premenstrual Syndrome) but more severe. For about 5% of women in the general population, this is experienced as a worsening mood during the days leading up to the menstrual cycle (Potter, Bouyer, Trussell & Moreau, 2009). These mood changes of depression, irritability, sadness, and anxiety can be as severe as chronic, ongoing, depressive or anxiety disorders and can have a significant impact on functioning.

### Did You Know?

- Women who experience PMDD can be at an increased risk for developing a Perinatal Mood and Anxiety Disorder (Amiel Castro, Pataky, & Ehlert, 2019).

- Women who have PMDD also often have an overlapping diagnosis of depressive or anxiety disorder (Pearlstein & Steiner, 2008; Buttner et al., 2013).

The connection between hormonal changes and mood are also seen in women who have difficult periods, such as heavy bleeding, for example. These women are at higher risk for postpartum depression (Muchanga, et al., 2017). And there is a similar correlation for women who have endometriosis. Are any of these part of your reproductive journey? As we talked about in Chapter 4, it's important to think about the various contributing risk factors for why you might be feeling the way you are.

## Postpartum Hormonal Changes and Risk for Depression And Anxiety Symptoms

After you had your baby, did you experience crying, abrupt mood changes, hot flashes, or feeling "out of sorts"? Immediately after having a baby, women don't often make the connection that there is a hormonal cause for their emotions, they just think something is wrong with them. Even though you may have seen other evidence of hormonal changes like your hair falling out, it can be hard to make the connection that hormonal changes are also impacting your mood. Following childbirth there are abrupt and significant changes in hormones that can make a woman vulnerable to symptoms of depression and anxiety. Some of these hormonal changes are shifts that occur in the levels of progesterone, estrogen, prolactin, cortisol, oxytocin, and thyroid hormones. Some symptoms of increased cortisol for example, that can occur after childbirth, are increased high blood pressure, flushed face, muscle weakness, increased thirst, and changes in mood like feeling down. Stress can also be a cause of increased cortisol release. (Hannibal & Bishop, 2014). While these hormonal changes and subsequent symptoms are normal, they can trigger worrying and negative thoughts, such as: "Because of my high blood pressure after giving birth I am afraid something really bad will happen to me," "I am not normally so emotional, why do I keep crying?" "Will this ever stop? I am just not myself."

As we discussed before, it is quite common for women to experience the onset of Perinatal Mood and Anxiety disorders during times of hormonal adjustments such as when starting birth control, when restarting menstruation after baby, and when weaning breastfeeding (Soares & Zitek, 2008). While most of these hormonal shifts cannot be avoided, it can be helpful to know about the impact of hormones on mood so that you can be aware and manage what you can during these times.

- **Birth control:** If you are starting or restarting birth control after having your baby, monitor your mood for the first several months to notice any changes. There are several free apps where you can track your mood, or you can track your mood on your phone calendar as well.

- **Breastfeeding/chestfeeding weaning:** If it is possible to do so, it is recommended to slowly wean versus abruptly wean when stopping breastfeeding/chestfeeding so you can manage the adjustment of hormonal changes.

- **Exercise:** Exercise and sunlight exposure can be beneficial activities to buffer against hormonal fluctuations. When you get your provider's OK to begin moving your body again, this can be something within your control.

- **Meditation/Relaxation practices:** While your hormonal changes may be out of your control, the benefits of meditation and relaxation practices (see Chapter 10) can help to physically calm you.

- **Managing your stress:** Chapter 5 on self-care gave a lot of suggestions for how to manage stress such as taking microbreaks, outsourcing for added help, etc.

- **Increasing your support system:** Decreasing the burden on you will help decrease your stress. While your hormones may still be changing, you can build your village of support to take away some of your tension.

- **Identify your negative thoughts:** This can be a great time to circle back to Chapter 7 to review what hormonal or physical changes you are experiencing and how this impacts your mood and thoughts. We suggest you pause and return to some of the activities in that chapter to identify any negative thoughts you might be having around your hormonal or physical changes.

**Of the action items listed above, which most stands out for you to address this week?**
Depending on what season of life you are in (pregnancy, early postpartum recovery, etc.), which change do you want to make or what do you want to address?

_____
_____
_____
_____
_____
_____

# D-MER

There are two great myths in life: 1) Twinkies last forever, and 2) breastfeeding is easy and magical for everyone. For some, breastfeeding IS easy and magical. For others, it is really difficult, or it may not be an option at all. There are also hormonal changes with nursing, and there is a particular phenomenon we'd like you to know about to feel empowered in case this happens to you.

Some women experience Dysphoric Milk Ejection Reflex (D-MER, for short) which is a feeling of depression, anxiety, sadness or self-reported heartache during the letdown period of breastfeeding. Women who experience D-MER specifically experience mood symptoms only around this specific time of breastfeeding. This phenomenon is thought to have a hormonal connection due to oxytocin and dopamine. When milk release is triggered, the oxytocin level rises and dopamine abruptly and briefly drops. (Uvnas-Moberg & Kendall-Tackett, 2018).

It is also important again to note that weaning is one of those times in which there are hormonal shifts and can trigger symptoms of depression and anxiety for some. While eventual weaning is unavoidable for women who are breastfeeding, it is important to be mindful of your mood and symptoms during this time.

# Activity:

Now that we've introduced some common physical and biological changes and how they impact mood, it can be helpful to reflect on how some of the changes and symptoms you've experienced may have impacted your thoughts and mood specifically. For example, panic can happen when we catastrophize our body symptoms, such as feeling shaky from low blood sugar and thinking it is something more serious. We explored this more thoroughly in our "Managing Thoughts" section in Chapter 7.

**Below, please check any physical symptoms you are having and any thoughts related to those physical symptoms**.
*Of course we understand that some physical sensations may be indicative of more serious issues, and we hope that you take good care of yourself and get them checked out with your doctor. The exercise below is a good way to connect your physical sensations with any beliefs and thoughts you are having so that you can better understand how thoughts and physical symptoms can be related.*

**Physical Symptoms**:

☐ Shakiness

☐ Increased heart rate

☐ Dizziness

☐ Lethargy (low energy)

☐ Nausea

☐ Stomach cramps

☐ Feeling flushed

☐ Change in appetite

☐ Headaches

☐ Blurred vision

☐ Spotting

☐ Other physical symptoms: _____

**Thoughts related to the physical symptoms:** (For example, "When my heart was racing, I totally thought I was having a heart attack and I was so scared," or "Every time I was nauseated I thought I wouldn't be able to handle it and it would never end!")

_____

_____

_____

_____

_____

**Ways my mood and thoughts are impacted by physical symptoms during pregnancy and the postpartum phase:** (For example: "When I am nauseated, I am so anxious, I won't leave the house" or "When I'm exhausted or have a headache, I'm worried I'll never feel like myself again.")

_____

_____

_____

_____

_____

_____

_____

_____

**Stress reducing or self-soothing activities I can engage in (check all that appeal to you or that you plan to do within the week):**

☐ Use a breathing technique to feel more centered and in control of my body (see Chapter 10 for suggestions). This is particularly helpful when nauseated, or feeling chest tightness or other body sensations.

☐ Practice a mindfulness technique such as the five-senses technique (see Chapter 10 for more information) to pay attention to what is around you, and draw attention away from your worrying mind.

☐ Engage in a relaxation technique (see Chapter 10 for ideas) such as a body scan or using a relaxation app for a brief meditation exercise.

☐ Take a slow walk, paying attention to the scenery around you.

☐ Take a bath (if medically cleared).

☐ Get a massage (if ok'd by your provider).

☐ Get a manicure or pedicure (even a non-professional DIY one counts!)

☐ Take a mommy and me exercise class (or do a free gentle at-home yoga class online briefly while baby is napping).

☐ Listen to calming music or a podcast that makes you happy.

☐ Use your favorite lotion or perfume just because it makes you feel good.

☐ Another self-soothing activity I can do this week: _____

_____

# Important Takeaways

- The most common times women experience mood disorders (or changes) are during times of hormonal fluctuations like menstruation, pregnancy, postpartum, starting birth control, weaning breastfeeding, and menopause.

- Some women experience Dysphoric Milk Ejection Reflex (D-MER, for short) which is a feeling of depression, anxiety, sadness, or self-reported heartache during the letdown period of breastfeeding.

- The hormonal changes you are experiencing during pregnancy or after having a baby may have an impact on your mood.

- Your hormonal and physical changes can also impact your sex drive.

- While some of your hormonal changes may be out of your control, there are many things in your control to help you manage your stress and mood better.Did You Know?

- The most common times of onset of mood disorders for women are:
- during menses
- during and after pregnancy
- with the first menstruation post-pregnancy
- when weaning breastfeeding
- during menopause (Soares & Zitek, 2008).

# CHAPTER 14

# A TOUGH SITUATION JUST GOT TOUGHER

## *HOW PARENTING A CHILD WITH HEALTH ISSUES CAN IMPACT YOUR MOOD*

Bethany Warren, LCSW, PMH-C
Beth Creager Berger, Ph.D.

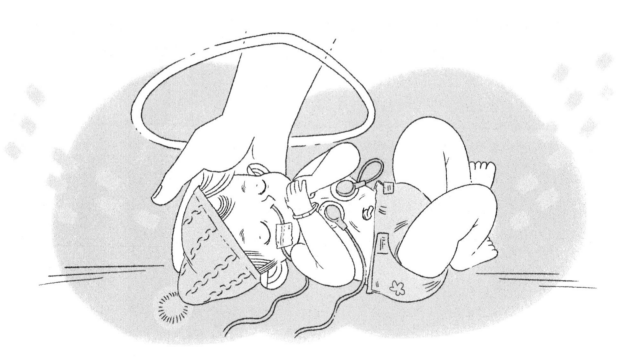

I want to put my hand out and touch you. I want to do for you and care for you. I want to be there when you're sick and when you're lonesome.

- *Ethan Frome*, by Edith Wharton

DOI: 10.4324/9781003144021-17

Did your baby spend time in the NICU? Does your child have a diagnosis of a disability, or was born with a medical issue that was scary during your pregnancy or early postpartum recovery period? All of these things can add on to the stress of postpartum adjustment and growing into your role as a parent, and of course, impact your mood in very significant ways. Research even shows us that this is the case, and if you are the parent of a child with *any* diagnosis (or even if your baby briefly needed extra care), you know how hard this is emotionally and what a toll this takes on your mental health. There are really no words to describe how scary it is to give birth and be told your baby needs to go into the NICU or that there might be an issue with your child that needs extra follow up. It is a club where no parent wants to be a member.

Nobody expects to leave the hospital without their child. No one's vision of their birth involves separation from their baby, whether it is for months or even hours. Understandably, moms with a baby in the NICU are 40 percent more likely than moms of healthy infants to experience depression, anxiety, and trauma symptoms (Tahirkheli, Cherry, Tackett, McCaffree & Gillaspy, 2014; Fowler, Green, Elliott, Petty & Whiting, 2019). There are many reasons these new moms are more susceptible to symptoms of depression and anxiety, none the least of which is fear of the unknown. "Will my child be ok?", "Will my child lead a normal life?", or "Will my child live?" might be thoughts you've had to face, and more. Having a sick baby is nothing anyone envisions, and new parents can feel completely derailed. You may also be experiencing a tremendous feeling of grief. You may be grieving the experience you thought you would have and the birth experience you had planned. You may be grieving the lack of "normalcy" and grieving what might have been. You may have had dreams of what this was supposed to be like, and your dreams are now having to be readjusted.

Whether your child was diagnosed with an acute, short-term issue (like a NICU stay for jaundice), or a chronic long-term health issue, we appreciate the range of emotions you may be feeling. You may have had time during your pregnancy to prepare for this diagnosis, or you may have learned at delivery that there were complications. Either way, this has been hard, and this is likely an unexpected journey. You are probably still finding ways to cope with an entirely different outcome than what you were expecting. The feeling of being out of control is often central in these situations. You may be frustrated with not being able to enjoy the small things you thought you would, like nursing your baby, or snuggling him in the way you imagined.

You may even have difficulty with hearing or saying the name of your baby's diagnosis or find many aspects of this triggering. We say this gently, honoring that you may still be early on in this journey. We hope to introduce you to tools and ideas that will help you navigate this new normal in a way to help you find some sense of ease in your situation, whatever that may be for you.

## Did You Know?

- Moms with babies in the NICU are more likely to suffer symptoms of anxiety, depression and trauma than moms of babies born without intervention.

- Mothers who deliver babies that require emergency intervention (such as resuscitation or going to the NICU) are at higher risk for trauma symptoms (Silverstein et al., 2019).

- Helplessness is a common feeling of parents with sick children.

## Guilt

Feeling guilty as a parent is really common, right? However, when is the last time your guilt told you anything important? Guilt is a common feeling, in particular, if you have a child with any health issues. But guilt does not provide us any value. When people feel guilty they may stew on the guilty thought for hours afterwards with really no helpful insights coming from feeling so bad. Many moms of sick children feel intensely guilty and responsible. "Did I do something to cause this?", "Could I have prevented this if I did something different during my pregnancy?", or "Am I being punished?" You might even be having a crisis of faith right now; we find this quite common with many of our clients. And, unfortunately, you may infer real or perceived blame from your loved ones around you who are asking questions about how this happened. If you have older children, you may feel incredibly pulled in numerous directions, and as a result, may feel guilty about not being as available to them at this time, and worried about the impact on them.

Holding on to guilt in this situation may be a way of finding control over this situation that feels out of your control. However, this type of guilt can be painful, and we encourage you to do everything you can to try and not go there. At the very least, if you can acknowledge the guilt thoughts by using the skills taught in Chapters 7 and 8, it can be useful to see how your thoughts may be impacting your emotions and mood. We wish that any of this was easy, but it is not and we can only offer you to do whatever you can to stay mindful and not create a false narrative of why you think this happened. In fact, you may feel better by focusing on what is in your control.

## What Is Within Your Control?

By focusing on activities that are within your control right now, you may feel more empowered. Examples include **(check all that you want to try this week if possible):**

- ☐ Find ways to care for your baby in whatever ways are permitted/possible, such as giving him a bottle, changing him, and being involved in his care.

- ☐ Hold your baby, if and when possible, so he can feel your touch.

- ☐ Talk quietly to your baby, letting her know she is safe and loved.

- ☐ Ask if you can play music or sing quietly to your baby.

- ☐ Spend time with your older children when you can (even brief moments of connection).

- ☐ Delegate one thing off of your to do list this week (e.g. preparing meals for your family).

- ☐ Get to know your baby's treatment team.

- ☐ Become as medically informed as you can by asking questions and doing research.

- ☐ To stay organized, you can use a notebook with a section for each specialist. Take notes from each appointment because it can be common to be forgetful and overwhelmed right now.

- ☐ Switch providers, if possible, if it does not feel like a good fit.

- ☐ Follow through with medical and therapeutic recommendations from doctors, physical and occupational therapists, etc.

☐ Connect with support groups or online communities with other parents.

☐ Seek professional support or treatment for yourself.

☐ Surround yourself with positive, informed, and optimistic people.

☐ Other things I can do to feel more in control _____

## Activity

**As you read above, guilt is really common so let's help you name any of your guilty thoughts. Remember that idea from Chapter 8 of naming your dragon so you can slay your dragon? List any guilty thoughts you may be having about your child.** (Examples might be: "Maybe I didn't take good enough care of myself", or "It's stressful to spend time in the NICU, I don't want to go right now", or "I'm not cut out for this.")

_____

_____

_____

_____

_____

**Remembering the lessons you learned from Chapters 7 & 8, how might you think about these thoughts another way? How might you talk back to these thoughts, or talk to a friend if she were saying this to you?** (For example: "Lots of people exercise in their pregnancy and their babies are fine", or "I bet lots of parents find the NICU stressful, I'm probably not the only one", or "I'm overwhelmed right now but I will get support to figure this out")

_____

_____

_____

_____

_____

If it was really difficult for you to think about healthier ways to talk to yourself, it's ok. You may be having a really hard time right now and could likely benefit from more support. Perhaps you could bounce what you're feeling off a friend, a loved one, or a therapist, and they can help you see things with a different perspective. **Who might you reach out to this week?**

_____

_____

_____

## You Are Not Alone

There are often support groups in the hospital for parents of NICU babies. Likewise, depending on your baby's medical issue, there are often many online groups where parents can share their fears and struggles with other parents who get it. Finding a support group or chat forum can be tremendously helpful for validation and resources. We've often found that sometimes "you have to kiss a couple of frogs before you get your prince," so to speak, when it comes to groups. You may have to try out a few groups before you find your people. You might also find that groups are not for you in this stage of your experience because it may be too difficult to hear about other peoples' stories. That is ok too.

## The Impact on Your Relationship

Having a child with a medical or disability diagnosis can be really difficult on your relationship with your partner. It is likely you are both stressed and overwhelmed right now and just doing your best. There may even be deeper resentments that are surfacing now, such as remembering disagreements about whether or not to have children, or fighting over feeling unsupported or unheard. When we are in fight-or-flight survival mode, we are not at our best, nor are we our most compassionate and empathetic selves. Communication can break down, and we can quickly become irritable and snappy at each other.

Try and talk to each other if you can. Nobody else understands what you are going through but your partner is the closest one who can try. This is a time to practice turning *toward* each other rather than **away**, even if it is hard to spend some energy investing in each other right now. A review of Chapter 9 and the impact on your roles changing and how you can communicate your needs can be helpful here.

**If you haven't already shared it, what is the one thing you would like your partner to know about how you are feeling?** (An example might be that you are feeling jealous about the time your partner spends at work, and while you understand he needs to keep working in order to feel normal, you need a break away from the house too).

_____

_____

_____

**What are you curious about regarding how your partner is feeling?** (An example might be that your partner is more silent about her emotions so sometimes you make assumptions that she doesn't care or isn't as worried as you are. You would like to know if that's the case and what she thinks about your son's upcoming surgery).

_____

_____

_____

**What is one thing you can each do for each other this week?** (Examples might be: having a mini date night where you go out to eat on the way home from the hospital, give each other some time off this week so you can each be alone for a bit, or each of you does the chore the other hates, etc.)

_____

_____

_____

## Trauma

Perhaps you had an emergency cesarean section and your baby was immediately whisked away to the NICU so she could be stabilized. Maybe there were unknown medical issues that presented themselves after delivery and you had to immediately become an expert, spending numerous nights at your baby's bedside, advocating for her, and reaching out to others for support and information. Maybe you learned about your baby's medical condition during your pregnancy and were faced with difficult decisions and scary, anxiety filled weeks. And perhaps you have a chronically ill child, where you are now frequently hypervigilant and aware of numerous dangers that can lurk around any corner. This is trauma, and the impact on you can be cumulative and significant. It is important to validate the traumatic experiences that you may have endured, or are still enduring, as the parent of a child with medical issues.

## Trauma Symptoms

As you may remember from learning about trauma symptoms in Chapter 3, it can be common to replay the events of your birth or your baby's hospitalization over and over. You may also be experiencing an increased sense of feeling unsafe, like you have to be on guard at all times, and on watch over your child now. This can be incredibly difficult and have an impact on the quality of your sleep, and your general mood. Parents who have gone through stressful childbirth and postpartum experiences can have posttraumatic stress reactions including irritability, increased tearfulness, nightmares, and even dissociation (feeling like either you or the situation is not real). There can also be a delayed onset of symptoms after the initial danger is over, like when the baby finally comes home from the NICU or has gone through her surgery. If this resonates with you, this chapter is here to help you address and manage your symptoms. We also review professional treatment options for reproductive trauma in Chapter 16 and provide suggestions in the Resources Chapter. Trauma can have an impact on your emotional, mental, and physical wellbeing, and can often make you feel out of control.

**This can be a helpful time to review ideas from page 134 to empower you to practice things that are within your control**.

*Alicia's pregnancy seemed like a textbook pregnancy; everything was fine until the delivery. And then during pushing, all of a sudden, her dream turned into a nightmare, and she had an emergency cesarean section because her team said her baby was in "fetal distress." It felt like something out of a movie. In fact, Alicia felt like she was watching the whole thing from far away. When she had her baby, they immediately whisked him off to the NICU so she never got to see or hold him for many hours. The first time she did, it didn't even feel like he was actually her son. It took several times of people telling her what was going on for her to understand the cardiac diagnosis they were explaining they had discovered, and it felt like she was out of her body. The next several weeks of visiting the NICU, tests, monitor alarms, procedures, and sleepless nights flew by. Slowly Alicia learned more about what her son was going through, and she felt more comfortable in that overwhelming environment. But then she got home with him a month later and felt herself really spiraling down mentally again. All the events seemed to replay over and over, and it was so scary to be on her own now without the monitors making sure her son's heart was fine. It wasn't until she joined an online support group for other moms of babies with cardiac issues and started therapy that she started to feel like she could manage this. When Alicia learned that she had experienced a lot of traumas, it helped her to understand why she was feeling the way she was. No wonder she felt so hypervigilant and on guard!*

## Involvement with Your Child's Medical Providers

Whether your child was born premature, or is having an ongoing health issue, it is likely you will have a slew of medical providers that you will be engaging with over the years. Some people are hesitant to speak up to their child's treatment team because they feel intimidated. However, YOU are a crucial part of your child's medical team. It's important for you to gain experience and confidence with asking about your child's care and learn how to become an advocate for him. What are ways you can speak to the medical staff in a way that is comfortable for you? Here is an example:

*"Hi Nurse, I have noticed my infant startles sometimes when she is sleeping. It is concerning to me and before I go Google about it, can you explain why this might be happening, or I would like the doctor to discuss this issue*

*with me so I can learn what this might be. Can you contact her and let me know when she is available to speak to me? Thank you so much I really appreciate it."*

It's ok to ask questions. It's ok to ask for clarification on things that you're confused about. It's even ok to switch providers if possible, if it's not a good fit. What questions might you have? **Some common questions might be (check which ones might pertain to you):**

☐  What is this test (treatment, procedure) that you are ordering?

☐  Why are you ordering this test?

☐  What are you looking for or trying to learn with this test?

☐  If this were your child, would you order this test?

☐  If this were your child, what questions would you want answered?

☐  How serious is my child's condition?

☐  What are the long-term consequences of this condition?

☐  What might come up next for my baby?

☐  What can I do to be a helpful part of my baby's care?

☐  What information would be helpful for me to know, or where can I learn more?

☐  Is it ok for me to leave right now to rest (pump, eat, etc.)? Will you contact me if I need to return?

☐  Another question I have is: _____

Planning ahead makes communication easier, particularly if you feel intimidated to ask questions or speak up. **How can you directly and effectively approach the medical staff? How can you ask questions you want answered?** (Refer back to Chapter 9 for more examples of direct communication which can be used with health professionals as well!)

_____

_____

_____

_____

_____

_____

Establishing a relationship with your baby's medical team can be a helpful way to increase your feelings of being in control and decrease feelings of anxiety. Please ask questions whenever you have them. You are not a burden, you are not being needy (we hear this worry a lot from our clients). It is OK for you to ask for clarification of your baby's health circumstances. Reaching out to the medical doctors, not "Dr. Internet" ensures you get correct information. The internet tends to create panic and anxiety in people because you might unintentionally land on a page with inaccurate information for your specific situation. If you are someone that likes to do your own research, we get it and recommend you stick with your medical team for answers and ask for additional reading suggestions and resources. We also recommend you ask your medical team if they can connect you with any parents of children with the same issue who might be willing to talk to you. This can be invaluable for support, information and connection. Lastly, don't hesitate to change doctors or medical providers if you feel you are not being heard or if they are not a good fit for you. It is often a good idea to get a second opinion anyway, if for nothing else than peace of mind.

## It Is Ok to Not Feel Ok

During this time so much is different than how you had planned. Suddenly, you are not able to care for your baby the way you had visualized. If your baby is still in the hospital, you may not be able to feed her as you had hoped or even dress or touch her because the nurses seem to be doing most of what you thought you would be doing. You may not have gotten to celebrate the baby's arrival with family and friends as you had pictured in your mind. Instead, many of your days have likely been in a hospital with fluorescent lights that confuse day and night as time runs by. You may have been further traumatized by the constant beeping and alarms that are there to alert doctors and nurses but instead have you on constant alert. You may have witnessed doctors and nurses running down the hall for a "code blue" and feel fear and sadness, yet relieved that it is not your child they are running towards. There are so many emotions you are experiencing all at the same time.

## Finding a Balance of Taking Care of Both Your Baby and You

Even if you are out of the hospital, your hypervigilance and protectiveness of your baby continues. Your focus understandably is on your baby but it is also incredibly important to also focus on your own self-care when you are able. You will feel like you can keep going and sustain the pace needed if you can take some care of yourself. Let's be honest, it is really hard to parent, period. But it is even harder if you are in a space of constant survival mode. What might you need in order to keep going? If you have not yet read Chapter 5 about self-care, this may be a good time to review those concepts.

### Small Steps Towards Feeling a Little Better Right Now:

- It is important that you make sure you are eating regularly and getting some sleep (this sounds simple but often goes out the window).
- It can be hard to do, but take breaks to move your body and get fresh air.
- It's important to rely on trusted family, and friends.
- Learning how to communicate with your medical providers and nurses will help you feel safer — learn their names, keep a binder to keep track of information.
- If you are at the hospital most of the day, ask a friend or family member to sit there instead sometimes so you can have some time to go home, shower, take care of yourself and even have a bit of time to yourself.

## Activity:

**Below is a list of common struggles when dealing with the stress of a child with a disability or a medical diagnosis. What are some small steps you can take to help you feel physically or mentally better?**

**Eating:** I could _____

**Family or friend support:** I could reach out to _____

**Time to self:** I could _____

**Community Support** (e.g. hospital or online groups) I could _____

**Connection with partner:** I could (e.g. hold hands, understand their pain too, discuss my needs)

_____

**Establish a relationship with the medical team:** I could

_____

## Parenting a Child with A Disability

All parents have hopes and dreams when pregnant. Upon the knowledge of being pregnant it is unlikely that anyone plans at that time for a child with any extra issues. Does the thought cross our minds? Sure. But we do everything we can to ensure we have a healthy child. We may change our diet, try meditation, and go to doctor's appointments. And somewhere along the way, we get the news that something is not quite right. So we readjust our plans and readjust our goals and readjust our dreams. And we grieve (which is normal).

Of course there is guilt when feeling grief or sadness because there are so many things for which we still feel thankful. It is understandable that you need time to adjust to the loss of your dream. You might also be grieving that your child will have a different life than the one you had dreamed of for her. We all want our children to lead a life with minimal struggles. Real talk: it is understandable to grieve the loss of the baby that you had hoped for just as you are falling in love with the baby you have. And you are sooooo tired. Exhausted from having to educate yourself about the disability, exhausted from coping with the physical and emotional demands of taking care of a child with extra needs, exhausted from a decrease in any personal time. Having a child with a disability or a diagnosis to attend to can also take attention away from other children in your family and interfere in your connection with your partner. Having a child with any diagnosis might reinforce your own fears of not fitting in with others. For example: "What if this diagnosis takes over our whole life?" or "What if I go to a play group and the other moms stare?" It definitely can be more challenging to have a child with a disability. Be gentle with yourself.

### Did You Know?

- Research shows that moms of children with disabilities are more at risk for having symptoms of depression and anxiety.

- 20%–30% of children in the United States have a chronic illness (Brown et al., 2008).

- So if you're identifying with this and noticing mood changes (or feeling more stressed), it's common and you're not alone!

**Circle any negative feelings you have been experiencing within the past two weeks related to parenting your child.**

**Sadness  Exhaustion  Guilt  Anger  Disbelief  Confusion**

**Shock  Loss of Focus  Anxiety  Fear  Denial  Other: _____**

**What do you need to help support you through this time? (Check all that interest you)**

☐ Time to yourself (reading a book, driving in your car, listening to a podcast, just sitting)

☐ Connection with others (phone calls, text, coffee with a friend, etc.)

☐ Doing a small pleasurable activity (doing your nails, exercise, listening to music, gardening…)

☐ Time with your partner

☐ Take a walk instead of doing a chore

☐ Watch a TV show

☐ Join a support group

☐ Help with older children

☐ Help with your baby so that you can spend alone time with your older children

☐ Expand your village of support

**What can you do to make any of these things happen?** (Examples include: call loved ones to keep you company, arrange with your partner so you can have time to yourself, look into ways to have respite care for your child, etc.)

_____

_____

_____

_____

_____

_____

## Important Takeaways

- Having a child with a medical issue or a disability can be incredibly difficult and can have an even greater impact on your mood.

- Parents with children with a disability or whose children are in the NICU have an increased risk of developing depression and anxiety.

- You may have experienced trauma which can have an added impact on your mood and emotional wellbeing.

- Having a child with a disability or medical issues can have an impact on your relationship as well.

- While all of these things may be out of your control and difficult, it can be helpful to focus on what is in your control: taking small steps towards self-care, building your support team, and learning how to navigate parenthood.

# Part IV
# What's Next?

# CHAPTER 15

# FROM AMBIVALENT TO TERRIFIED AND EVERYTHING IN BETWEEN

## *CREATING AN EMPOWERING POSTPARTUM PLAN FOR THE NEXT PREGNANCY*

Bethany Warren, LCSW, PMH-C
Beth Creager Berger, Ph.D.

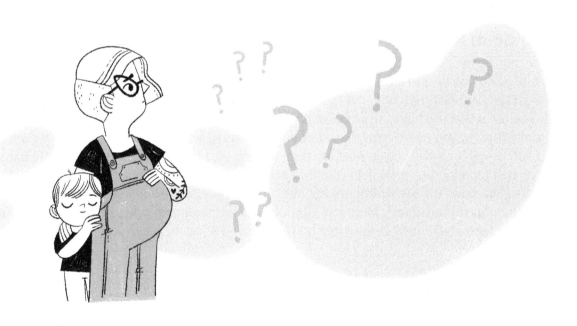

I may not be where I want to be but I'm thankful for not being where I used to be.

- Habeeb Akande

DOI: 10.4324/9781003144021-19

We get it. If you are still in the middle of your Perinatal Mood and Anxiety symptoms, or just starting to feel like yourself again, the thought of having another baby might bring about a lot of fear. We know that the thought of conceiving again and the potential of going through this again can be terrifying. As humans, we are really good at avoiding suffering. If we have just touched a hot stove and burned ourselves, we are smart at not returning to that same hot stove.

However, as Perinatal Mental Health therapists, we also know that this is quite a complex issue because many of you DON'T want to conceive again because you might be fearful of having a Perinatal Mood and Anxiety Disorder (or difficult mood symptoms) again but you may have always dreamed of having more than one child. Or, you may just be exhausted and the thought of doing this again is inconceivable (no pun intended, haha!). It is important to look at the real risks versus perceived risks of having another baby as well as learn how to manage those risks.

---

**Did You Know?**

- By having a prior PMAD you are anywhere between 25% and 41% higher risk of developing PMAD symptoms with a subsequent pregnancy (Wisner et al., 2004).

- However, those numbers only tell us that women are at higher risk. They do not tell us about the course, duration and intensity of a woman's experience the next time.

---

## The Good News:

While we do not want to minimize this risk of developing mood symptoms (or a PMAD) again, what we can tell you as practitioners is that being prepared is crucial. One good thing of having gone through this before is that you have learned so much about yourself and about how to help yourself! Even without realizing it, you have learned some of your mood triggers (such as lack of sleep or difficulty with breastfeeding), or what you needed for support (and didn't have). You also learned what you could have used more of (like meal deliveries and postpartum recovery support), and less of (isolation from others). You have also learned that these mood symptoms are treatable and you can get better! What we will do in this chapter is help you formulate a pregnancy and postpartum plan for a subsequent pregnancy using your own experience and wisdom as well as our own.

## Why A Pregnancy and Postpartum Plan?

Working on a pregnancy and postpartum plan can help minimize the risks of developing a PMAD and managing the symptoms if they do actually occur again. It can help you feel empowered and in control. Whether or not you ultimately move forward toward conceiving is of course your choice, and working with a therapist on this further can be a great use of some therapy sessions. We recognize this is a complex issue and for some, choosing *not* to have another baby feels empowering, too.

*Prisha had pretty difficult Obsessive-Compulsive symptoms after the birth of her first baby. It took her a long time of attending therapy and taking medication before she started to feel better. It was a really tough decision to take medication because her family did not understand not only what she was going through, but also the need for medication. So, by the time she got help and got better, it had been a long process. The thought of getting pregnant again with even the smallest chance of going through this whole mental health storm again was so overwhelming! Prisha's family lives so far away and she doesn't have much support nearby. She felt so isolated, and the thought of managing this again felt like a lot. But yet she and her husband always wanted two children, so it was a tough bind to be in. With the help of Prisha's therapist, they worked on a plan together to prepare for her next pregnancy. It felt like such a relief to create tangible steps that felt in her control when the rest of her mental health was still somewhat unpredictable. Prisha's husband even joined a few sessions so he could voice his concerns and help participate in the planning. He had some great suggestions and they finally felt empowered for whenever they decided to move forward.*

Let's work together now to think of you and your family's needs during this vital recovery time. We created this postpartum plan inspired by one developed by DONA International (DONA.org). You can custom design it to fit your specific needs. You can find more information to help you with your postpartum planning in our Resource chapter.

## Activity

**As you think back to your pregnant or postpartum mood changes, what are some of the crucial things you were lacking?** (Ideas might be breastfeeding support, professional support during your vital "fourth trimester" recovery time, support at night, meals from others, mental health resources, etc.)

_____

_____

_____

_____

_____

Now let's go through some common planning needs and see what is relevant for you. Not all of these will pertain but it can be easier to be prepared.

**1. How to manage your mental health next time:** As you think back to your experience with mood changes, what do you wish you knew? Maybe your symptoms were missed by one of your providers, you had difficulty reaching out to others for help, or you had difficulty identifying that something was wrong for quite a while.

**Who would you reach out to if you felt "off" next time during your pregnancy or postpartum recovery** (for example your partner, your doula, a good friend, your obstetrician or midwife, your therapist, someone in your community, etc.)?

_____

_____

_____

_____

Even though every pregnancy and postpartum recovery period can be different, it can be helpful to think about HOW you might know you were feeling differently.

**Jot down some ideas here of how you might notice you were struggling** (for example: "I was isolating from others" or "I wasn't sleeping at night when the baby was sleeping" or "it was a struggle for me to take care of myself in addition to the baby.")

_____

_____

_____

_____

**What would you do differently this time to manage those struggles?** (For example, "If I was not sleeping, I would ask for help from a family member, hire a postpartum doula ASAP or start a sleep swap schedule with my partner", or "If I was noticing depressive symptoms, I would seek out therapy much sooner").

_____

_____

_____

_____

And finally, as you have worked your way through this workbook (and possibly with the help of a mental health provider and/or a support group), our hope is that you have built a treatment team around you. List those people below so that for your next pregnancy you can easily remember who you can reach out to for help, if needed. **We always recommend a few visits with a mental health provider throughout the pregnancy and at least one to two visits in the early postpartum period for mothers who have had a prior experience with a PMAD or serious mood changes** (from the standpoint of support and checking in). Remember, with treatment you will get better, and you are not alone!

**The people on my mental health team and safe people who I can go to for professional treatment, planning, or support include:**

_____

_____

_____

_____

2. **How you can protect your sleep next time:** Sleep is really important as you've likely discovered. As you have learned, new parents need extra help to ensure they get as much rest and sleep as possible and this is even more important when your mood is off. Your sleep was likely affected by your mood symptoms and vice versa. Whether you were having difficulty falling back asleep due to racing thoughts after feeding the baby, or feeling like no amount of sleep was enough in addressing your poor energy and lack of motivation, your sleep likely took a big hit.

   Whether or not you experience Perinatal Mood and Anxiety symptoms again, sleep support is helpful. Having people available to help you get better sleep at night and for naps during the day can feel life changing. We recommend that you schedule this type of support for several weeks postpartum and you can always cancel it if you find you don't need help after all. This would be a great time to start problem solving on how you can further build your village of support.

**The following people could be available to help us get our rest:**

☐ Postpartum night doulas

☐ Family members

☐ Friends

☐ Neighbors

☐ Members of my community groups

☐ Members of my religious community

☐ Other support people: _____

**A sleep schedule we can try to follow next time would be:** (For example: I do the last feeding at night, my partner does the middle feeling and I get up early in the morning)

_____

_____

_____

3. **Feeding yourself:** How often did you find yourself missing meals or eating your kid's goldfish crackers for dinner on the fly? Regular and healthy meals and hydration are important to help keep your mood stable. Preparing ahead can help you avoid skipping meals and enable others to help you prepare for your baby and be a part of your village.

**Things I can do to ensure I am getting enough nutrition throughout the day:**

☐ Ask friends, family, neighbors or community members to bring you meals

☐ Ask friends to start a meal train or meal delivery service as a baby shower gift

☐ When people ask you "what can I do?", let them know what types of foods you like and what specific meals you would enjoy

☐ Prepare _____ number of frozen meals before you deliver, ideally

☐ Compile a list of your favorite take-out and delivery options

☐ Other options: _____

4. **Feeding your baby:** Whether or not feeding your baby was stressful for you and contributed to your mood symptoms, it's likely you have already thought about how you would like to feed your baby if you had another pregnancy. Whether you hope to breastfeed/chestfeed exclusively, bottle-feed using formula or pumped breast milk or a combination of the two, you've likely put a lot of thought into this. It can be useful to plan now for support for when you actually start enacting your plan once you transition home after your delivery.

**What did you experience last time? Check some nursing struggles you may have encountered:**

☐ Sore nipples

☐ Mastitis

☐ Low milk supply

☐ Low birthweight

☐ Judgment from others (for example if you wanted to stop nursing)

☐ Guilt about the amount of time you breast/chestfed

☐ Difficulty latching

☐ Exclusively pumped

☐ Trauma around nursing

☐ Other: _____

**If you bottle, pumped, cup or tube fed your baby, or used another means of feeding your baby other than breast/chestfeeding, check any struggles you may have encountered:**

☐ Difficulty with allergies

☐ Difficulty with supply

☐ Judgment or lack of support and understanding from others

☐ Finding the right formula or donor source

☐ Other: _____

You may have had some struggles with feeding your baby. Women often internalize these difficulties (i.e. "I've failed") which leads to shame and guilt. Whether or not you choose to breastfeed/chestfeed it can be helpful to seek out support to help you through this, such as a lactation consultant, doula, friends, aunts, etc.

Similarly, if you have chosen to pump and bottle-feed your baby or use formula, it's important that your support people know that this is your choice so that they can empower and support you!

**The following friends, professionals or relatives are supportive of my preference of how to feed my baby:**

_____

_____

_____

_____

_____

5. **Who is in your village?** Having someone to talk to who can empathize with our experiences normalizes our problems and makes them more bearable. We all need validation, right? Friends who have children can become a part of your circle by enhancing your life and building on your existing support network. If you don't yet have friends with young babies, then think about where you might start making these friends. Suggestions include postpartum support groups, childbirth education classes, music classes, prenatal/postnatal fitness classes, breastfeeding support groups, friends of friends, cousins or siblings with children, and play groups.

**I've identified these people as part of my village in Chapter 9:**

_____

_____

_____

_____

**Some ideas for further building your village of support, such as new friends and people who have young children can include the following:** (suggestions can be found in our Resources chapter)

_____

_____

_____

_____

6. **How to handle sibling adjustment:** You are likely worried about the impact another baby would have on your older children, and are potentially scared to rock the boat. We hear it all the time in our practices that moms are worried they will never love another baby like they did their first, or scared they will mess everything up by bringing in another baby. You are not alone in any of these thoughts! It's normal and healthy for the older siblings to experience an adjustment when a new baby comes home.

**Ways you can help ease the transition on your older child(ren) might include (check all that might apply):**

☐ Maintain a daily routine for them as much as possible.

☐ Ask your friends or family to spend special one-on-one time with them, or give you breaks so that you can have that time.

☐ A small gift from the new baby to the older sibling is something that can also help your older sibling to feel excited by the new baby (some people might call this bribery but we like to call it positive reinforcement).

☐ Ask for friends or family to give you breaks by providing tangible help (such as driving your children to school, etc.).

☐ Practice continuing one special ritual or time of day with your older child (such as bath time, bedtime book reading, etc.) while the other partner swaps out with the baby.

☐ Other things you can do: _____

7. **Last but certainly not least, how to protect your relationship with your partner:**

   If you are in a relationship, it is important to carve out couple time with your partner. "Couple time?" you may ask as you roll your eyes. "Couple time? What the heck is that?" The relationship you have with your partner is foundational. It needs to be a priority. Your relationship and the lack of quality time with each other may have been a source of stress for you with your first baby and contributed to your symptoms. As we explored in Chapter 9, there have likely been changes to your relationship since becoming parents, and time together can help you reconnect.

**Ways that we can reconnect include (check all that apply):**

☐ Asking friends, professionals or family for breaks so that we have time together

☐ Maintaining small rituals together that are still feasible (such as watching our favorite TV show at night or taking walks on the weekend)

☐ Doing small gestures of touch for connection throughout the day

☐ Telling your partner things that you appreciate about him/her

☐ Text or call to connect through the day when you are apart

☐ Other activities that we enjoy together and are relatively easy to do as new parents:

_____

## Important Takeaways

- Research tells us that by having a PMAD you are at anywhere between 25% and 41% higher risk of developing PMAD symptoms with a subsequent pregnancy (Wisner et al., 2004).

- It can be important to have a plan for a subsequent pregnancy to minimize any of these risk factors and help you feel empowered and in control!

- By learning from your last experience, you can think of what you needed more of, less of, what were triggers to your mood changes, and plan accordingly.

- However, those numbers only tell us that women are at higher risk. They do not tell us about the course, duration and intensity of a woman's experience the next time.

# CHAPTER 16

# SO WHAT NOW?

## *TREATMENT OPTIONS*

Bethany Warren, LCSW, PMH-C
Beth Creager Berger, Ph.D.

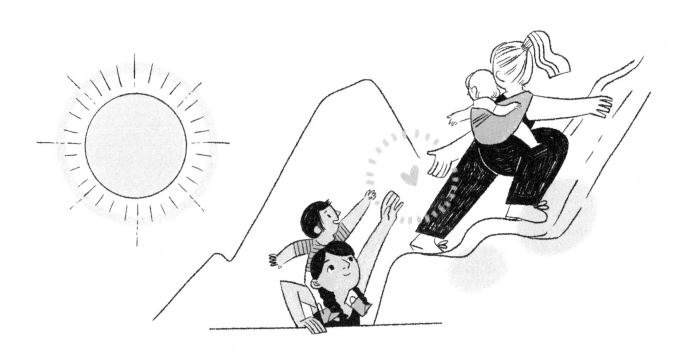

Isn't it funny how day by day nothing changes, but when you look

back everything is different?

- *Prince Caspian*, by C.S. Lewis

DOI: 10.4324/9781003144021-20

## What Else Can I Do?

This workbook has been chock full of strategies to help you feel better. You have learned a lot of skills to manage your symptoms. We know how hard this has been; working on yourself when you're feeling bad takes a lot of effort! Perhaps you have seen significant improvement and would like to continue to work on yourself. If you would like to keep working on building skills, we wanted to review additional treatment options that you can explore – knowledge is power!

Remember, these symptoms during the perinatal period are treatable and you do not need to suffer. You especially do not need to suffer alone. Hopefully you have noticed some improvement, or at a minimum, the edge has been taken off as you feel armed with some tools to manage your symptoms. We will go through some of the additional treatment options below, and similarly to an "a la carte menu", we encourage you to pick and choose which options sound good to you. Refer to our list of resources at the end of the book to help you find help in your area.

## How Do You Know If You Need Professional Help?

You don't have to have something serious going on to benefit from therapy. Anyone can benefit from therapy. In fact, you may find that you want to find a therapist to help you manage your perinatal moods, even if they are quite mild, simply because parenting is tough! This stage of life is a major disruption to your "normal", and it can be really nice to have time to yourself with a sympathetic listener.

However, is important to get professional help if you are experiencing any of the following:

- Serious symptoms that are impacting your functioning (see Chapter 2 for a review of more serious symptoms if you need a refresher)

- Urges to harm yourself, your baby, or anyone else require immediate help. As a reminder, here are numbers you can access, or go to your closest Emergency Room:

**US National Suicide Hotline 1-800-273-8255**
**UK Samaritans Crisis Line 116 123**
**Text HOME to 741741 to connect with a crisis counselor in the US and Canada, 85258 in the UK, and 50808 in Ireland**.

So, let's talk about therapy, and all of the different options. We wanted to briefly explain some of these therapy orientations to give you an overview of what your therapist may offer you if you seek out therapy with a counselor who specializes in Perinatal Mental Health.

## Psychotherapy

Psychotherapy or counseling helps give a different perspective and build coping skills to help you through this challenging time. It's time just for you that is so rare during this season of life as a new parent! Therapists that specialize in the perinatal period are often open to you bringing your baby or toddler with you, if you prefer.

## Did You Know?

- There are many different types of individual psychotherapy that are effective for Perinatal Mood and Anxiety Disorders

- These include Cognitive Behavioral Therapy (CBT), EMDR therapy, Dialectical Behavioral Therapy (DBT), psychodynamic, family systems therapy, and Interpersonal Therapy (IPT) among others.

- Regardless of the type of therapy, if you are not feeling well, it is important to get help so you can begin to feel better!

**Cognitive Behavioral Therapy (CBT)** is one type of therapy that has been studied extensively in the treatment of depression and anxiety and has been shown to be helpful in up to 80% of patients who utilize it (Butler & Beck, 2000; DiMauro et al., 2013). We taught you some skills from this therapy in Chapter 7 and 8 and how to apply them to perinatal symptoms. CBT is often brief and solution focused. A focus of CBT is to change maladaptive thinking patterns or thoughts and behaviors in order to promote a change in mood.

**EMDR therapy** is a type of psychotherapy originally created and extensively studied specifically for trauma, but now also been shown to be effective for depression, anxiety, grief, loss, eating disorders and other psychological issues (Shapiro, 2001; Bisson & Andrew, 2007). EMDR therapy is also helpful for Perinatal Mental Health, particularly when there are traumatic issues such as a distressing birth experience, infertility, pregnancy loss or negatively held beliefs that cannot be shaken, such as "I'm a bad mother", "I failed", or "I'm powerless" (van Deursen-Gelderloos & Bakker, 2015; Baas, van Pampus, Braam, Stramrood, & de Jongh, 2020)

**Dialectical Behavioral Therapy (DBT)** focuses on two opposite forces – acceptance and change. When a person can accept their experience, they then can more easily change the behaviors that do not serve them. For example, if you are able to accept that you are struggling with anxiety (rather than deny and fight your reality), it will be easier to address your avoidance behaviors, such as not going out with your baby to public spaces. DBT essentially helps you deal with overwhelming emotions (Linehan, 1993). The core areas of focus with DBT are learning emotional regulation skills, skills for managing distress and crisis, interpersonal effectiveness skills (communication, etc.), and mindfulness. These skills are all profoundly helpful for a new parent experiencing mood or anxiety symptoms.

**Exposure and Response Prevention (ERP)** is a type of cognitive behavioral therapy to help decrease the frequency and severity of distress caused by obsessive thoughts and compulsive behaviors. A person is slowly exposed to their fears in order to reduce their distress, while learning how to avoid engaging in compulsive behaviors. This work is paired with learning relaxation techniques to lower distress.

**Interpersonal Psychotherapy (IPT)** has also been shown to be effective for Perinatal Mood and Anxiety Disorders (Grigoriadis & Ravitz, 2007) as it addresses some of the core themes of parenthood such as role changes, interpersonal conflicts (including how to learn how to communicate more effectively), and building support. You learned some great IPT skills in Chapter 9.

## Activity:

**Of the various therapies we just talked about, which ones most caught your eye? Which ones do you find yourself most attracted to, and why?**

_____

_____

_____

## Couples Therapy

Do you find yourself more irritable at your partner, blaming him or her for anything that goes wrong? Do you find yourself with a hair trigger response, or, on the flip side, walking on eggshells around your partner? Has this been a tough transition, feeling like your partner isn't compassionate or tuning into your needs? Do you feel like they just don't get you anymore?

### Did You Know?

- Remember, up to 67% of couples report marital dissatisfaction after the birth of a baby (Gottman, 2007).

- This can increase even further when one of the partners is experiencing a PMAD.

Do you remember how we talked about how common PMADs are in dads and same sex partners? If you AND your partner are both experiencing mental health symptoms, conflict might be sky-high in your house right now in addition to going through the typical strain of just learning how to be parents together. As it is, parenting is difficult enough, but going through a mental health crisis together can put a strain on how you communicate with each other, the roles you've taken on in your family, and even your values and goals.

This can be a difficult time for the family unit and can even have an impact on other members of the family, such as other children, other extended family members, and even pets who can now go ignored! This can be a good opportunity for couples therapy to help strengthen your foundation, learn some new communication skills, and help give you tools to navigate through this phase. Couples therapy can help you feel like this is a shared issue and your partner can be empowered to take a role in your treatment as well. Couples therapy can be incredibly beneficial for mood changes because partner support has a measurable effect on women experiencing any symptoms around this time (Misri, Kostaras, Fox, & Kostaras 2000). It can be useful to find couples therapists who specialize in Perinatal Mental Health AND couples work. Many therapists are open to having the baby in session with you.

## Support Groups

How often are you telling yourself, "Everyone else is better at doing this than I am!" or "I am such a bad mom"? It can be so validating to hear another mom speak about her experience and have it echo your own. Support groups can be a valuable resource to new parents for many reasons. They can provide education, support, stress reduction techniques, and cognitive therapy techniques to help give new parents a different perspective. New parents can feel validated with the realization they are not alone. It's also a great way to meet and connect with other new parents!

It is important that new parent groups allow you to bring your baby with you in order to increase the likelihood of participation. Ideas for support groups you could attend include postpartum support groups led by therapists, support groups facilitated by peers, breastfeeding support groups, religious groups, and new parent playgroups where the support is secondary to socialization. If you go to a support group and find that the members are just simply "not your people", don't give up! Most areas have several different support groups and you can often try another group to see if there is a better fit. Like a group of friends, it can be important for it to feel comfortable to open up to new people.

## Medication

Often, new moms do not want to take medication if they are pregnant or nursing for fear of the potential harm to the baby. We get that this is a complicated decision. How often do you hear the phrase "I don't even want to take a Tylenol!" regarding medication while pregnant or breastfeeding? It is important to look at the big picture regarding risk, and inform yourself with reliable information (not just Dr. Internet!) and also consider the impact of NOT being treated. Questions like: "How am I functioning?", "How is my ability to take care of myself and my baby?", and "How long have my symptoms (or impairment in functioning, etc.) been going on?" can be useful self-prompts.

It is important to remember that when parents get treatment and start to feel better, the baby benefits as well. The question becomes: what do you need to improve your functioning?

It is important to weigh all of the above while making this difficult decision, and to have a prescriber (a psychiatrist, psychiatrist nurse practitioner, ObGyn or primary care physician) who has experience prescribing medication for pregnancy and postpartum issues and who can help answer ALL of your questions and concerns and review any relevant studies with you. Resources to find providers and education will be at the end of the book. Even if you are undecided, it can be useful to have an appointment with a prescriber with perinatal experience so you can weigh your options, empower yourself with knowledge and learn about medications that are possible with pregnancy and nursing.

Some women are surprised that it can take a few weeks or longer to notice the benefit of medication and some of our clients have admitted to us that they wish they had made the decision to start medication sooner. However, we understand it's a personal decision. Some of your mood symptoms can be treated without medication while using other forms of treatment. If other forms of therapy are not working as fast as you had hoped, medication can be a viable option. There is no need to suffer through the pain of this. You deserve to be happy and you deserve to begin to enjoy your child and your life.

## Intensive Outpatient Programs (IOPs)

For those that are needing more frequent appointments, or finding they need more structured support, there are IOPs. IOPs often meet anywhere between three to five times a week, and are a mix of individual psychotherapy and support groups. Some also provide medication management by a psychiatrist if indicated. These programs are highly structured and supportive, meet during the day for several hours, and often last several weeks with the goal of stabilizing the person until they feel able to step back down into once-a-week therapy. Reasons for mothers seeking IOPs might include those who are feeling so anxious or depressed, or those who are having frequent intrusive and racing thoughts so much that they need additional support and structure. Some women who are really struggling with a lack of motivation and having a difficult time getting through each day find IOPs especially beneficial. Women struggling with suicidal thoughts also find the safety and routine of IOPs helpful. There are some IOPs that welcome babies as part of the program.

## Self-Care

We discussed a lot of self-care throughout this book and we encourage you to continue thinking about what you need to practice for self-care on a regular basis. Go back and review the self-care chapter (Chapter 5) and notice some of the themes you took away. Write them below with some of the biggest "takeaways" from this workbook: **What do you want to keep working on? What skills have you learned that you will keep practicing?**

_____

_____

_____

_____

_____

_____

## Utilizing Support

Expanding your village is crucial as a new parent, but even more so if you are dealing with mental health issues. This can be difficult for every woman, because let's face it, it can be hard to approach strangers, ask for help, or make ourselves vulnerable by sharing when we are not doing well. As women, we are not often taught how to be vulnerable and how to receive help, as many of us identify as caregivers and are honored to take care of others' needs first. This is an important season for you because it is a season of receiving help. As a new mother, you are in a season of learning to care for a newborn, yourself as a new mother, and your newly growing family. How might you learn how to access support in a way that feels comfortable for you?

_Claudia was really great at taking care of everybody in her life. She was a caring daughter and wife, and was known as the neighbor that takes care of everyone else's needs first. She's the go-to person when someone is sick, or needs to carpool, or needs to borrow something. So when Claudia started noticing she was feeling off, she was so scared. It was hard enough to feel depressed because she was fearful she may never feel like herself again. But it was even harder to think about having to admit to others that she might need help. So at first she kept up a brave front and kept cooking, taking care of herself and everyone around her with the same level of intensity. But then she noticed she was drained, getting more resentful and irritable, and really sad. She just wanted someone to take care of her but it was so hard to ask! So she started small. She asked her neighbor to go on a walk with her and bravely told her she was struggling. And it went so well! Her neighbor was so kind, and told her that she went through postpartum stuff too, and that it will get better. Her neighbor ended up being so sweet and kept checking on her, and even brought her some meals! It felt weird being on the receiving end of care, but also really nice. Claudia was really glad she reached out._

## Activity:

What's great about building our village is that we don't have to start from scratch and that we can expand from the resources that we already have. We already helped you identify some of your support here and build more on this concept in the chapter on expanding your support (Chapter 9).

**Who is already in your village? And who have you more recently included into your village?**
This might include trusted family members, friends, neighbors, people from your religious community or hired professionals (doulas, therapists, lactation consultants, etc.)

_____

_____

_____

_____

## Activity:

**Of all of the treatment options that we listed throughout this chapter, what is the most realistic to choose right now in the short term?**

_____

_____

_____

_____

**Of all of the treatment options that we listed throughout this chapter, what sounds interesting but is something that you might consider more in the long term?** What additional information or resources might you need in order to help you make this decision?

_____

_____

_____

_____

**What are any potential hurdles to getting the help that you've identified?** Examples might include finding someone that takes your insurance, finding the time or energy to make calls, overcoming the internal beliefs you might have about treatment (i.e. "therapy isn't for me, it's for other people"), etc.

_____

_____

_____

_____

**With all of the skills that you have learned, how might you overcome any of these hurdles?** (Examples can include: asking a friend for a therapist recommendation, scheduling a time to make calls, calling a provider from one of the organizations listed in the Resource Chapter, etc.)

_____

_____

_____

_____

### Remember:

- You are not alone.
- Mood changes during the pregnancy and postpartum period are really common and are temporary.
- This will change.
- You are the best parent for your baby!

You have now made it through this workbook and we are so proud of you! We imagine you have made some significant progress, perhaps in how you feel, or maybe in how you look at yourself and the symptoms you are feeling. You are now armed with information and resources, and we applaud you. You've got this.

## Important Takeaways

- There are many different types of individual psychotherapy that are effective for Perinatal Mood and Anxiety Disorders and symptoms.

- Support groups can be a valuable resource for this time in your life for education, support, validation, and to help you meet and connect with other parents!

- Medication can be a viable option for many parents to address their symptoms, and it is important to work with a prescribing provider who has experience with pregnant and postpartum women, and is well versed with the latest research in this field.

- You have worked so hard throughout this workbook and we are so proud of you! You have likely learned a lot about yourself and made progress with your symptoms. This chapter and the resources chapter gives you some additional ideas of what you can do next. You've got this!

# RESOURCES

*All of these resources are up to date by the time of publishing, so please check to ensure both the link and resource are still accurate! Also, of course this list is not exhaustive by any means but represents some good resources for support.*

## Websites

### Black Mothers:

- Black Mamas Matter: blackmamasmatter.org (Resources, Advocacy for Black Mothers, supporters of the Black Maternal Mental Health week)

- Shades of Blue Project: shadesofblueproject.org (Online support groups, resources, advocacy for Black mothers)

### Dads/Partners:

- Mayo Clinic Information about depression: mayoclinic.org/diseases-conditions/depression/in-depth/depression/art-20045943 (Information about supporting a family member or friend)

- Postpartum Dads: Postpartumdads.org (Stories, support, resources, blog posts)

- Postpartum Support International: postpartum.net/get-help/resources-for-fathers/ (Support for fathers, online chat forums)

- Postpartum Support International: postpartum.net/get-help/queer-parents/ (support for LGBTQ+ parents, and queer parents support group)

- Same-Sex Parents: same-sexparents.com (Support, education, resources)

### Expectant Mothers

- AIMS UK: aims.org.uk (Pregnancy and birth information in the UK, information about maternity care)

- Mothers and Babies Program: mothersandbabiesprogram.org (online or in-person Cognitive Behavioral Therapy course for expectant and new parents)

### EMDR Therapy:

- EMDR International Association: emdria.org (Information about EMDR therapy, finding a therapist by specialty type and geographic area)

## Emergency Resources:

- Crisis Text Line: crisistextline.org (Text HOME to 741741 to connect with a crisis counselor in the US and Canada, 85258 in the UK, and 50808 in Ireland.)

- HopeLine UK: papyrus-uk.org 0800 068 4141(practical advice on suicide prevention)

- Lifeline Northern Ireland: lifelinehelpline.info 0808 808 8000 (Referrals for therapy, mentoring, 24/7 suicide prevention)

- Mind: 0300 123 3393 (Infoline in the UK for mental health referrals, treatment options, advocacy services)

- National Suicide Prevention Lifeline: suicidepreventionlifeline.org/ 1-800-273-8255 (US lifeline available 24/7 for referrals and support)

- SAMHSA: Substance Abuse and Mental Health Services Administration samhsa.gov 1-800-662-4357 (US national helpline available 24/7 for referrals and information)

## General Perinatal Resources:

- Climb Out of the Darkness: postpartum.net/join-us/climbout/ (The world's largest event raising money and awareness about PMADs)

- DONA International: dona.org/ (How to find a doula, postpartum plans)

- MGH Center for Women's Mental Health: womensmentalhealth.org (Information about medication, studies/research, PMADs, treatment resources, etc.)

- PANDAS: pandasfoundation.org.uk (Postnatal Depression Awareness and Support in the UK, support groups, free hotline 0808 1961 776)

- Perinatal Anxiety and Depression Aotearoa: pada.nz/postnatal-depression/ (Support, information and access to treatment in New Zealand, 04 461 6318 / 021 024 82123)

- Perinatal Mental Health Project: pmhp.za.org (Support, information and access to treatment in South Africa, free helplines in English and Afrikaans)

- Postpartum Depression Kenya: ppdkenya.com/ (Awareness, Support and access to treatment in Kenya, free help at 254 733 424 361)

- Postpartum Stress Center: postpartumstress.com (Education, support, trainings, and treatment in the Pennsylvania area)

- Postpartum Health Alliance: postpartumhealthalliance.org (San Diego area, access to resources such as postpartum support groups, referrals to providers who specialize in PMADs, educational and training events, free warmline 619–254–0023, awareness and more)

- Postpartum Support International: postpartum.net (International connections to online support groups, referrals to providers worldwide who specialize in perinatal mental health, information, free helpline 1-800-944-4773, awareness and more)

- Postpartum Support Network Africa: postpartumafrica.org/ (Support, awareness and connections to treatment across Africa, 234 803 324 0575)

- Seleni Institute: seleni.org (Education, trainings and treatment in the NY area)

## Intensive Outpatient Programs:

To find the most updated list of Inpatient and Intensive Outpatient Perinatal Psychiatric Programs, please go to Postpartum Support International here: postpartum.net/get-help/intensive-perinatal-psych-treatment-in-the-us/

## Medication:

- Mother to Baby: mothertobaby.org/ (Medications and More during Pregnancy and Breastfeeding)
- Postpartum Support International Directory: psidirectory.com/listing/psychiatry-medication (Finding a Perinatal Psychiatrist, Nurse Practitioner, or other prescriber in your area)

## OCD:

- International OCD Foundation iocdf.org (Includes Information about Perinatal OCD)
- Maternal OCD: maternalocd.org/ (Resources for mothers and professionals, helpline for support, articles and research, UK based)

## Perinatal Advocacy:

- Blue Dot Project: thebluedotproject.org (National Symbol for Maternal Mental Health survivors, blogs, resources, advocacy)
- Every Mom Counts: everymothercounts.org (Advocacy to make pregnancy and childbirth safe for everyone, everywhere)
- 2020Mom: 2020mom.org (National US Maternal Mental Health Advocacy)

## PTSD/Birth Trauma:

- Birth and Trauma Support Center: birthandtraumasupportcenter.org/ (Peer support, resources for parents and professionals, referrals to providers)
- Birth Trauma Association: birthtraumaassociation.org.uk (Support, resources, information for parents and providers, birth stories, etc. UK based)
- Prevention and Treatment of Traumatic Birth: pattch.org (Education to prevent or reduce reproductive PTSD and promote effective treatments for recovery)
- Solace for Mothers after Traumatic Birth: solaceformothers.org (Support and resources for parents and professionals, online forums)

## Support or Parenting Groups:

- Peanut app: peanut-app.io (support and connection during fertility and becoming parents)
- Postpartum support groups in your area: postpartum.net/get-help/locations/united-states/ (International groups are also available)

- Same Sex parent support groups: familyequality.org/family-support/national-network-lgbtq-family-groups/ (parent support groups)

- Specific play groups: meetup.com (a way to meet other parents in your area including: single mothers, working mothers, stay-at-home fathers, etc.)

# Phone Apps

## Perinatal Mood and Anxiety Disorders:

- Moment Health: momenthealth.io/ (For UK parents: resources, mood tracker, connection to community)

- MGH Perinatal Depression Scale: itunes.apple.com/us/app/mghpds/id1239621118?mt=8 (Edinburgh Postnatal Depression Scale, access and linkages to resources)

- Veeda mom: apps.apple.com/us/app/veedamom/id1109489586 (Support during pregnancy and the first month after birth).

## Meditation/Relaxation/Breathing:

- Breathe2Relax: apps.apple.com/us/app/breathe2relax/id425720246 (Breathing techniques including diaphragmatic breathing)

- Calm: www.calm.com/ (Meditation and guided relaxation exercises including sleep stories)

- Headspace: headspace.com/headspace-meditation-app (Meditation exercises)

- Insight Timer: insighttimer.com/ (Free relaxation and guided meditation exercises including for sleep)

- The Mindfulness App: themindfulnessapp.com/ (Mindfulness and guided meditation exercises)

## Mood:

- Daylio play.google.com/store/apps/details?id=net.daylio&hl=en_US (mood tracker)

- CBT thought diary apps.apple.com/us/app/cbt-thought-diary/id1010391170 (Mood, CBT, and gratitude journal)

- SAM - Self Help for Anxiety Management: apps.apple.com/us/app/self-help-for-anxiety-management/id666767947 (self-help skills to manage anxiety)

# Podcasts

- First2Years: first2yearspodcast.com/postpartum-depression-pmads-what-who-the-path-to-help/ (Podcast Episode on PMADs and resources)

- Healthy Births, Happy Babies with Dr. Jay Warren: drjaywarren.com/podcast-3/ (Parenthood, fatherhood, supporting mom through her pregnancy and postpartum journey, PMADs, etc.)

- Mom and Mind momandmind.com/ (various Perinatal Mental Health topics including PMADs, pregnancy loss, birth trauma)

- New Mommy Media: pregnancymagazine.com/podcasts/delayed-postpartum-depression-symptoms (Various parenting topics including several Perinatal Mental Health episodes on PMADs, delayed depression after having a baby, self-care, relationships and "postpartum depression".

# Books

### Anxiety and Obsessive-Compulsive Disorder:

- *The Anxiety and Phobia Workbook* by Edmund J. Bourne

- *Cognitive Behavioral Therapy for OCD* by David Clark

- *The OCD Workbook: Your Guide to Breaking Free from Obsessive-Compulsive Disorder* by Bruce Hyman

- *Brain Lock* by Jeffrey M. Schwartz

- *Overcoming Unwanted Intrusive Thoughts: A CBT-Based Guide to Getting Over Frightening, Obsessive, or Disturbing Thoughts* by Sally M. Winston, Psy.D., and Martin N. Seif, Ph.D.

- *The Pregnancy and Postpartum Anxiety Workbook: Practical Skills to Help You Overcome Anxiety, Worry, Panic Attacks, Obsessions, and Compulsions* by Pamela S. Weigartz and Kevin L. Gyoerkoe

### Breastfeeding:

- *Before The Letdown: Dysphoric Milk Ejection Reflex and the Breastfeeding Mother* by Alia Macrina Heise

- *Latch: A Handbook for Breastfeeding with Confidence at Every Stage* by Robin Kaplan, M.Ed., IBCLC

### Cognitive Behavioral Therapy:

- *Feeling Good* by David Burns

- *Mind Over Mood* by Dennis Greenberger and Christine Padesky

- *Ten Days to Self Esteem* by David Burns

### Dads:

- *Factoring in Fathers* by Jane Honikman and Daniel Singley, Ph.D.

- *Fathering Right from the Start* by Jack Heinowitz

### Mindfulness and Relaxation:

- *Full Catastrophe Living* by Jon Kabat-Zinn

- *The Relaxation and Stress Reduction Workbook* by Martha Davis, Elizabeth Eshelman and Matthew McKay

### Parenthood:

- *The Fourth Trimester: A Postpartum Guide to Healing Your Body, Balancing Your Emotions, and Restoring Your Vitality* by Kimberly Ann Johnson

- *The Girlfriend's Guide to Surviving the First Year of Motherhood: Wise and Witty Advice on Everything from Coping with Postpartum Mood Swings to Salvaging Your Sex Life to Fitting into that Favorite Pair of Jeans* by Vicki Lovine

- *The Mother Dance: How Children Change Your Life* by Harriet Lerner

- *Mothering the New Mother: Women's Feelings and Needs after Childbirth* by Sally Placksin

- *Mother Nurture* by Rich Hanson, Ph.D., Jen Hanson, L.A.c., and Ricki Pollycove, M.D.

- *Operating Instructions: A Journal of My Son's First Year* by Anne Lamott

- *Everyday Blessings: The Inner Work of Mindful Parenting* by John Kabat-Zinn

- *Parenting from the Inside Out: How a Deeper Self-Understanding Can Help You Raise Children Who Thrive* by Daniel J. Siegel, M.D. and Mary Harzell, M.Ed.

## Perinatal Mood and Anxiety Disorders:

- *Beyond the Blues* by Shoshana S. Bennett, Ph.D. and Pec Indman, Ed.D., MFT

- *Down Came the Rain: My Journey Through Postpartum Depression* by Brooke Shields

- *Dropping the Baby and Other Scary Thoughts* by Karen Kleiman and Amy Wenzel

- *Good Moms Have Scary Thoughts: A Healing Guide to the Secret Fears of New Mothers* by Karen Kleiman, MSW

- *Inferno: A Memoir of Motherhood and Madness* by Catherine Cho

- *The Mother-to-Mother Postpartum Depression Support Book* by Sandra Poulin

- *The Postpartum Husband* by Karen Kleiman

- *This Isn't What I Expected: Overcoming Postpartum Depression* by Karen R. Kleiman and Valerie D. Raskin

## Relationship After Baby:

- *And Baby Makes Three* by John Gottman, PhD and Julie Schwartz Gottman

- *When Two Become Three: Nurturing Your Marriage After Baby Arrives* by Mark E. Crawford

## Same Sex (Female) Parents:

- *And Baby Makes More* by Susan Goldberg and Chloë Brushwood Rose

- *If These Ovaries Could Talk: The Things We've Learned About Making an LGBTQ Family* by Jaimie Kelton & Robin Hopkins

- *What's in a Name? Perspectives from Non-Biological and Non-Gestational Queer Mothers* by Emily Regan Wills, Raechel Johns, Sherri Martin-Baron

## Trauma/PTSD:

- *Birth Trauma: A Guide for You, Your Friends and Family to Coping with Post-Traumatic Stress Disorder Following Birth* by Kim Thomas

- *The Body Keeps the Score* by Bessel Van der Kolk, MD

- *Traumatic Childbirth* by Cheryl Tatano Beck, Jeanne Watson Driscoll, Sue Watson

# REFERENCES

Alcott, L.M. (2011). *Little Women*. Boston: Little, Brown & Company. (Original work published 1880.) Retrieved from Project Gutenberg: www.gutenberg.org/ebooks/37106

American Psychiatric Association (2004). *Practice guidelines for the treatment of patients with acute stress disorder and posttraumatic stress disorder.* Arlington, VA: American Psychiatric Association Practice Guidelines.

American Psychiatric Association (2013). *Diagnostic and statistical manual of mental disorders* (5th ed.). Arlington, VA: Author.

Amiel Castro, R. T., Pataky, E. A., & Ehlert, U. (2019). Associations between premenstrual syndrome and postpartum depression: A systematic literature review. *Biological psychology*, 147, 107612. https://doi.org/10.1016/j.biopsycho. 2018.10.014

Anderson, C. (2010). Impact of traumatic birth experience on Latina adolescent mothers. *Issues in Mental Health Nursing, 31*, 700–707.

Baas, M.A.M, van Pampus, M.G., Braam, L, Stramrood C.A.I., & de Jongh, A. (2020). The effects of PTSD treatment during pregnancy: systematic review and case study. *European Journal of Psychotraumatology*, 11(1), DOI: 10.1080/20008198.2020.1762310

Barba-Müller, E., Craddock, S., Carmona, S., Hoekzema, E. (2019). Brain plasticity in pregnancy and the postpartum period: links to maternal caregiving and mental health. *Arch Womens Ment Health* 22, 289–299. https://doi. org/10.1007/s00737-018-0889-z

Barney, L., Griffiths, K., Jorm, A., Christensen, H. (2006). Stigma about depression and its impact on help-seeking intentions. *Australian & New Zealand Journal of Psychiatry, 40* (1), 51–54.

Beardslee, W.R., Versage, E.M., Gladstone, T.R. (1998). Children of affectively ill parents: a review of the past 10 years. *J Am Acad Child Adolesc Psychiatry*. 37(11):1134–1141. doi:10.1097/00004583-199811000-00012

Beardslee, W. R., Bemporad, J., Keller, M. B., & Klerman, G. L. (1983). Children of parents with major affective disorder: A review. *The American Journal of Psychiatry, 140*(7), 825–832. https://doi.org/10.1176/ajp.140.7.825

Beck, C. (1995). Screening methods for postpartum depression. *Journey of Obstetric, Gynecological & Neonatal Nursing, 24(4)*, 308–12. https://doi.org/10.1111/j.1552-6909.1995.tb02481.x

Beck, C.T., Driscoll, J.W., Watson, S. (2013). *Traumatic Childbirth*. New York: Routledge.

Beck, A.T., Rush, A.J., Shaw, B.F., & Emery, G. (1979). *Cognitive therapy of depression*. New York: Guilford Press.

Berk, M., Sanders, K.M., Pasco, J.A., et al. (2007). Vitamin D deficiency may play a role in depression. *Med Hypotheses*. 69(6): 1316–1319. doi:10.1016/j.mehy.2007.04.001

Bernard-Bonnin, A.C. (1990). Canadian Pediatric Society, & Mental Health and Developmental Disabilities Committee. Maternal depression and child development. *Pediatrics and Child Health, 9*(8), 575–583.

Bisson, J., & Andrew, M. (2007). Psychological treatment of post-traumatic stress disorder (PTSD). *Cochrane Database of Systematic Reviews*, Issue 3. Art. No.: CD003388. DOI: 10.1002/14651858.CD003388.pub3.

Blustain, R. (2018, July 13). The Paradox of Postpartum Depression. Colorlines. www.colorlines.com/articles/ paradox-postpartum-depression

Bornstein, M.H. (2012). Caregiver responsiveness and child development and learning: From theory to research to practice. *Infant/Toddler Caregiving: A Guide to Cognitive Development and Learning,* ed. P.L. Mangione, 2nd ed. Sacramento: California: Department of Education.

Brown, G.W. & Moran, P.M. (1997). Single mothers, poverty and depression. *Psychological Medicine, 27* (1) 21–33.

Brown, R.T., Weiner, L., Kupst, M., Brennan, T., Behrman, R., & Compas, B.E. (2008). Single parenting and children with chronic illness: An understudied phenomenon. *Journal of Pediatric Psychology, 33,* 408–421.

Buck, K., Zekri, S., Nguyen, L., & Ogar, U.J. (2019). Cognitive behavior therapy for postpartum depression. *Am Fam Physician,* 100(4): 244–245.

Buttner, M., Mott, S.L., Pearlstein,T., Stuart, S., Zlotnick, C., & O'Hara, M.W. (2013). Examination of premenstrual symptoms as a risk factor for depression in postpartum women. *Arch Womens Ment Health,16*(3): 219–225.

Burns, David (1980). *Feeling good: The new mood therapy.* William Morrow and Company.

Burns D.D., Beck A.T. (1978). Cognitive Behavior Modification of Mood Disorders. In: Foreyt, J.P., Rathjen, D.P. (eds) *Cognitive Behavior Therapy.* Springer, Boston, MA. https://doi.org/10.1007/978-1-4684-2496-6_5

Centers for Disease Control (2008). Prevalence of self-reported postpartum depressive symptoms—17 states, 2004–2005. *Morbidity and Mortality Weekly Report,* 57(14), 361–366.

Centers for Disease Control (CDC). Diabetes During Pregnancy. Retrieved October 21, 2019. www.cdc.gov/reproductivehealth/maternalinfanthealth/diabetes-during-pregnancy.htm

Charuvastra, A., & Cloitre, M. (2008). Social bonds and posttraumatic stress disorder. *Annual review of psychology, 59,* 301–328. https://doi.org/10.1146/annurev.psych.58.110405.085650

Clark, D.M., Salkovskis, P.M., Hackmann, A., Wells, A., Ludgate, J., Gelder, M. (1999). Brief cognitive therapy for panic disorder: a randomized controlled trial. *J Consult Clin Psychol,* 67(4): 583–589. doi:10.1037//0022–006x.67.4.583

Cleaveland, C. & Frankenfeld, C. (2019). "They Kill People Over Nothing": An Exploratory Study of Latina Immigrant Trauma, *Journal of Social Service Research,* DOI: 10.1080/01488376.2019.1602100

Cosmi, E., Fanelli, T., Visentin, S., Trevisanuto, D., & Zanardo, V. (2011). Consequences in infants that were intrauterine growth restricted. *J Pregnancy.* 2011:364381. doi:10.1155/2011/364381

Cox, J.L., Holden, J.M., & Sagovsky, R. (1987) Detection of postnatal depression. Development of the 10-item Edinburgh Postnatal Depression Scale. *Br J Psychiatry, 150*: 782–786. doi:10.1192/bjp.150.6.782

Crenshaw, K. (1989) Demarginalizing the Intersection of Race and Sex: A Black Feminist Critique of Antidiscrimination Doctrine, Feminist Theory and Antiracist Politics. *University of Chicago Legal Forum,* 1989(1): 139–167.

D'Amico, Christine (2004). *The pregnant woman's companion: nine strategies that work to keep your peace of mind through pregnancy and into parenthood.* Attitude Press, Inc.

de Divitiis, A. M. (2016). Note sheet for pregnant women: EMDR group therapy protocol for the prevention of birth trauma and postpartum depression. In M. Luber (ed.), *Eye movement desensitization and reprocessing (EMDR) therapy scripted protocols and summary sheets: Treating anxiety, obsessive-compulsive, and mood-related conditions* (pp. 389–396). New York, NY: Springer Publishing Co.

Dimeo, F., Boller, M., Varahram, I., Proest, G., Halter, U. (2001). Benefits from aerobic exercise in patients with major depression: a pilot study. *British Journal of Sports Medicine, 35*(2): 114–117.

DiMauro, J., Tolin, D.F., Domingues, J., & Fernandez, G. (2013). Long term effectiveness of CBT for anxiety disorders in an adult outpatient clinic sample: A follow-up study. *Behaviour Research and Therapy,* 51(2): 82–86.

Dobson, K.S. (1989). A meta-analysis of the efficacy of cognitive therapy for depression. *Journal of Consulting and Clinical Psychology, 57* (3): 414–419.

DONA.org Postpartum Plan Retrieved from www.dona.org/wp-content/uploads/2016/12/postpartum-plan-template.pdf

Ellis, S.A., Wojnar, D.M., & Pettinato, M. (2014). Conception, pregnancy, and birth experiences of male and gender variant gestational parents: it's how we could have a family. *J Midwifery Women's Health,* 60(1): 62–69.

Fairbrother, N., Janssen, P., Antony, M.M., Tucker, E., & Young, A.H. (2016). Perinatal anxiety disorder prevalence and incidence. *Journal of Affective Disorders, 200,* 148–155.

Field, T., Morrow, C., Adlestein, D. (1993). Depressed mothers' perceptions of infant behavior. *Infant Behav Dev., 6*: 99–108.

Forgash, C., Leeds, A., Stamrood, C. & Robbins, A. (2013). Case Consultation: Forgash, C. (2000). When a PTSD Survivor Becomes Pregnant: Implications for EMDR Treatment. Retrieved from www.advancededucationalproductions.com/

Forgash, C., Leeds, A., Stramrood, C., & Robbins, A. (2013). Case Consultation: Traumatized Pregnant Woman. *Journal of EMDR Practice and Research, 7(1),* 45–49.

Fowler, C., Green, J., Elliott, D., Petty, J., Whiting, L. (2019) The forgotten mothers of extremely preterm babies: A qualitative study. *J Clin Nurs.,* 28(11–12): 2124–2134. doi:10.1111/jocn.14820

Gaynes, B.N., Gavin, N., Meltzer-Brody, S., Lohr, K.N., Swinson, T., Gartlehner, G., Brody, S. & Miller, W.C. (2005). Perinatal depression: prevalence, screening accuracy, and screening outcomes. *Evid Rep Technol Assess (Summ)* (119): 1–8. doi:10.1037/e439372005–001

Giardineeli, L., Innocenti, A., Benni, L., Stefanini, M.C., Lino, G., Lunardi, C., Svelto, V., Afshar, S., Bovani, R., Castellini, G., & Faravelli, C. (2012). Depression and anxiety in perinatal period: prevalence and risk factors in an Italian sample. *Archives of Women's Mental Health, 15* (1) 21–30.

Gopnik, A., Meltzoff, A.N., & Kuhl., P.K. (2009). *The Scientist in the Crib: Minds, Brains, and How Children Learn.* New York: HarperCollins.

Gottman, J.M., Gottman, J.S. (2007). *And Baby Makes Three: The Six-Step Plan for Preserving Marital Intimacy and Rekindling Romance After Baby Arrives.* Danvers, MA: Harmony Books.

Graw, P., Recker, S., Sand, L., Kräuchi, K., Wirz-Justice, A. (1999). Winter and summer outdoor light exposure in women with and without seasonal affective disorder. *J Affect Disord. 56(2–3):* 163–169. doi:10.1016/s0165–0327(99)00037–3

Greenberger, D., Padesky, C. (1995). *Mind Over Mood: A Cognitive Therapy Treatment Manual for Clients.* New York: Guilford Press.

Grigoriadis, S., & Ravitz, P. (2007). An approach to interpersonal psychotherapy for postpartum depression focusing on interpersonal changes. *Can Fam Physician, 53*(9), 1469–1475.

Hall, E. & Steiner, M. (2013). Serotonin and female psychopathology. *Women's Health, 9(1):* 85–97.

Hammen, C., Burge, D., Burney, E., Adrian, C. (1990). Longitudinal study of diagnoses in children of women with unipolar and bipolar affective disorder. *Arch Gen Psychiatry, 47(12):*1112–1117.

Hammen, C., Gordon, D., Burge, D., Adrian, C., Jaenicke, C., Hiroto, D. (1987). Maternal affective disorders, illness and stress: Risk for children's psychopathology. *Am J Psychiatry,144:* 736–41.

Hannibal, K.E., Bishop, M.D. (2014). Chronic stress, cortical dysfunction and pain: a psychoneuroendocrine rationale for stress management in pain rehabilitation. *Physical Therapy (94)* 12; 1816–1825.

Hegel, M.T., Ferguson, J. (1997). Psychophysiological assessment of respiratory function in panic disorder. *Psychosomatic Medicine, 59* (3): 224–230.

Hendric, V., Altshuler, L.L., Suri, R. (1988). Hormonal changes in postpartum and implications for postpartum depression. *Psychosomatics, 39*(2): 93–101.

Henshaw, C. (2003). Mood disturbance in the early puerperium: a review. *Arch Womens Mental Health, 6:* S33–S42.

Herrell, H.E. (2014). Nausea and vomiting of pregnancy. *American Family Physician, 89* (12): 965–970.

Hölzel, B.K., Carmody, J., Vangel, M., Congleton, C., Yerramsetti, S.M., Gard, T., & Lazar, S.W. (2011). Mindfulness practice leads to increases in regional brain gray matter density. *Psychiatry research, 191*(1), 36–43.

Huang, L., Zhao, Y., Qiang, C., & Fan, B. (2018). Is cognitive behavioral therapy a better choice for women with postnatal depression? A systematic review and meta-analysis. *PloS one, 13*(10), e0205243. https://doi.org/10.1371/journal.pone.0205243

Hughes, H. (2008). Management of postpartum loss of libido. *Journal of Family Health Care, 18*(4): 123–125.

Hugo, V. (1994). *Les Misérables.* I. Hapgood, Trans. New York, NY: Thomas Crowell & Co. (Original work published 1887.) Retrieved from Project Gutenberg: www.gutenberg.org/files/135/135-h/135-h.htm

Hutcheon, J.A., Lisonkova, S., Joseph, K.S. (2011). Epidemiology of pre-eclampsia and the other hypertensive disorders of pregnancy. *Best Pract Res Clin Obstet Gynaecol., 25*(4): 391–403.

Jannati, N., Mazhari, S., Ahmadian, L. (2020). Effectiveness of an app-based cognitive behavioral therapy program for postpartum depression in primary care: A randomized controlled trial. *International Journal of Medical Informatics, 141,* 104145. https://doi.org/10.1016/j.ijmedinf.2020.104145

Jung, V., Short, R., Letourneau, N., & Andrews, D. (2007). Interventions with depressed mothers and their infants: modifying interactive behaviours. *Journal of affective disorders, 98*(3), 199–205. https://doi.org/10.1016/j.jad.2006.07.014

Kjeldgaard, H.K., Vikanes, Å., Benth, J.Š., Junge, C., Garthus-Niegel, S., & Eberhard-Gran, M. (2019). The association between the degree of nausea in pregnancy and subsequent posttraumatic stress. *Archives of women's mental health, 22*(4), 493–501. https://doi.org/10.1007/s00737-018-0909-z

Kleiman, K. (2019). *Good Moms Have Scary Thoughts: A Healing Guide to the Secret Thoughts of New Mothers.* Familius LLC.

Kleiman, K. & Raskin, V.R. (2013). *This isn't what I expected: overcoming postpartum depression*. Boston, MA: Da Capo Press.

Ko, J.Y., Rockhill, K.M., Tong, V.T., Morrow, B., & Farr, S.L. (2017). Trends in Postpartum Depressive Symptoms—27 States, 2004, 2008, and 2012. *Morbidity and Mortality Weekly Report, 66*: 153–158. http://dx.doi.org/10.15585/mmwr.mm6606a1External.

Kozhimannil, K.B., Trinacty, C.M., Busch, A.B., Huskamp, H.A., & Adams, A.S. (2011). Racial and ethnic disparities in postpartum depression care among low-income women. *Psychiatric services, 62*(6), 619–625. https://doi.org/10.1176/ps.62.6.pss6206_0619

Landau, J. & Saul, J. (2004). Facilitating family and community resilience in response to major disaster. In F. Walsh & M. McGoldrick (eds), *Living beyond loss* (pp. 285–309). New York: Norton.

Lara-Cinisomo, S., Wisner, K.L., Burns, R.M., & Chaves-Gnecco, D. (2014). Perinatal depression treatment preferences among Latina mothers. *Qualitative health research, 24*(2), 232–241. https://doi.org/10.1177/1049732313519866

Lazar, S.W., Kerr, C.E., Wasserman, R.H., Gray, J.R., Greve, D.N., Treadway, M.T., McGarvey, M., Quinn, B.T., Dusek, J.A., Benson, H., Rauch, S.L., Moore, C.I., & Fischl, B. (2005). Meditation experience is associated with increased cortical thickness. *Neuroreport, 16*(17), 1893–1897.

Lee, A., Lam, S., Sze Mun Lau, S., Chong, C., Chui, H., & Fong, D. (2007). Prevalence, course, and risk factors for antenatal anxiety and depression. *Obstetrics and Gynecology, 110*(5), 1102–1112.

Lewis, C.S. (1951) *Prince Caspian: The Return of Narnia*. Stuttgart: Macmillan Company.

Linehan, M.M. (1993). *Cognitive-behavioral treatment of borderline personality disorder*. New York: Guilford Press.

Lyons-Ruth, K., Connell, D., Grunebaum, H., Botein, S. (1990). Infants at social risk: Maternal depression and family support services as mediators of infant development and security of attachment. *Child Dev. 61*: 85–98.

Main, M. (1996). Overview of the field of attachment. *Journal of Consulting and Clinical Psychology 64* (2): 237–43.

Markman, H.J., Floyd, F., Stanley, S., & Lewis, H. (1986). Prevention. In N. Jacobson & A. Gurman (eds), *Clinical handbook of marital therapy* (pp. 173–195). New York: Guilford Press.

McLearn, K.T., Minkovitz, C.S., Strobino, D.M., Marks, E., Hou, W. (2006). Maternal depressive symptoms at 2 to 4 months postpartum and early parenting practices. *Archives of Pediatric and Adolescent Medicine, 160*: 279–284.

Misri, S., Kostaras, X., Fox, D., Kostaras, D. (2000). The impact of partner support in the treatment of postpartum depression. *Can J Psychiatry, 45*(6): 554–558.

Mott, S.L., Schiller, C.E., Richards, J.G., O'Hara, M.W., & Stuart, S. (2011). Depression and anxiety among postpartum and adoptive mothers. *Archives of women's mental health, 14*(4), 335–343. https://doi.org/10.1007/s00737-011-0227-1

Muchanga, S., Yasumitsu-Lovell, K., Eitoku, M., Mbelambela, E.P., Ninomiya, H., Komori, K., Tozin, R., Maeda, N., Fujieda, M., Suganuma, N., & Japan Environment and Children's Study Group (2017). Preconception gynecological risk factors of postpartum depression among Japanese women: The Japan Environment and Children's Study (JECS). *Journal of Affective Disorders, 217*, 34–41. https://doi.org/10.1016/j.jad.2017.03.049

Mulcahy, R., Reay, R.E., Wilkinson, R.B., Owen, C. (2010). A randomised control trial for the effectiveness of group interpersonal psychotherapy for postnatal depression. *Arch Womens Ment Health, 13*, 125–139. https://doi.org/10.1007/s00737-009-0101-6

Murray, L., Fiori-Cowley, A., Hooper, R., & Cooper, P. (1996). The impact of postnatal depression and associated adversity on early mother–infant interactions and later infant outcome. *Child development, 67*(5), 2512–2526.

NICHD Early Child Care Research Network (1999). Chronicity of maternal depressive symptoms, maternal sensitivity, and child functioning at 36 months. *Developmental psychology, 35*(5), 1297–1310.

Nickerson, M. (ed.) (2017). *Cultural competence and healing culturally based trauma with EMDR therapy: Innovative strategies and protocols*. New York, NY: Springer.

O'Hara, M. & Wisner, K. (2014). Perinatal Mental Illness: Definition, Description, and Aetiology. *Best Practice & Research Clinical Obstetrics & Gynaecology, 28* (1), 3–12.

O'Hara, M., Stuart, S., Gorman, L, & Wenzel, A. (2000). Efficacy of Interpersonal Psychotherapy for postpartum depression. *Archives of General Psychiatry, 57 (11)*, 1039–1045.

Paulson, J.F., & Bazemore, S.D. (2010). Prenatal and postpartum depression in fathers and its association with maternal depression. *JAMA, 303* (19) :1961–1969.

Pearlstein, T., Steiner, M. (2008). Premenstrual dysphoric disorder: burden of illness and treatment update. *Journal of Psychiatry & Neuroscience, 33*(4): 291–301.

Pope, C.J., Oinonen, K., Mazmanian, D., Stone, S. (2017). The hormonal sensitivity hypothesis: A review and new findings. *Medical Hypotheses*,102, 69–77. doi.org/10.1016/j.mehy.2017.03.012.

Potter, J., Bouyer, J., Trussell, J., Moreau, C. (2009). Premenstrual syndrome prevalence and fluctuation over time: Results from a French population-based survey. *Journal of Women's Health 18*(1): 31–39.

Rados, S.N., Marijas, M., Andelinovic, M., Cartolovni, A., & Ayers, S. (2020). The role of posttraumatic stress and depression symptoms in mother–infant bonding. *Journal of Affective Disorders, 268* (1): 134–140.

Rosenkranz, M.A., Davidson, R.J., Maccoon, D.G., Sheridan, J.F., Kalin, N.H., & Lutz, A. (2013). A comparison of mindfulness-based stress reduction and an active control in modulation of neurogenic inflammation. *Brain, behavior, and immunity*, 27(1), 174–184. https://doi.org/10.1016/j.bbi.2012.10.013

Ross, L.E., Steele, L., Goldfinger, C., & Strike, C. (2007). Perinatal depressive symptomatology among lesbian and bisexual women. *Archives of women's mental health*, 10(2), 53–59. https://doi.org/10.1007/s00737-007-0168-x

Russell, E.J., Fawcett, J.M., Mazmanian, D. (2013). Risk of obsessive-compulsive disorder in pregnant and postpartum women: a meta-analysis. *J Clin Psychiatry*, 74(4): 377–385.

Schwartz, J.M. (2016). *Brain Lock: Free Yourself from Obsessive-Compulsive Behavior. 20th anniversary ed.* New York: Harper Perennial.

Seaburn, D., Landau-Stanton, J., & Horwitz, S. (1995). Core intervention techniques in family therapy process. In R.H. Mikesell, D.D. Lustermann, & S.H. McDaniel (eds). *Integrating family therapy: Handbook of family psychology and systems theory* (pp. 5–26). Washington, DC. American Psychological Association.

Shapiro, F. (2001). *Eye movement desensitization and reprocessing: Basic principles, protocols and procedures* (2nd ed.). New York: Guilford Press.

Silverstein, R.G., Centore, M., Pollack, A., Barrieau, G., Goplan, P., & Lim, G. (2019). Postpartum psychological distress after emergency team response during childbirth. *Journal of Psychosomatic Obstetrics and Gynaecology*, 40(4): 304–310. doi: 10.1080/0167482X.2018.1512095.

Skalkidou, A., Hellgren, C.M., Comas, W., Sylvein, Poromaa, I.S. (2012). Biological aspects of postpartum depression. *Women's Health, 8 (6)*: 659–672.

Sockol, L.E. (2015). A systematic review of the efficacy of cognitive behavioral therapy for treating and preventing perinatal depression. *J Affect Disord*. 177: 7–21. doi:10.1016/j.jad.2015.01.052

Soares, C.N. & Zitek, C. (2008). Reproductive hormone sensitivity and risk for depression across female life cycle: A continuum of vulnerability? *Journal Psychiatry Neuroscience, 33*(4): 331–343.

Solomon, Z. (1990). Does the war end when the shooting stops? The psychological toll of war. *Journal of Applied Social Psychology, 20*:1733.

Somerville, S., Dedman, K., Hagan, R., Oxnam, E., Wettinger, M., Byrne, S., Coo, S., Doherty, D., & Page, A.C. (2014). The Perinatal Anxiety Screening Scale: development and preliminary validation. *Archives of women's mental health*, 17(5), 443–454. doi.org/10.1007/s00737-014-0425-8

Spinelli, M. (2017). *Interpersonal Psychotherapy for Perinatal Depression: A Guide for Treating Depression During Pregnancy and the Postpartum Period* (2nd edn). CreateSpace Independent Publishing Platform.

Stuart, S. & Robertson, M. *(2012). Interpersonal Psychotherapy: A Clinician's Guide.* (2nd edn) CRC Press.

Tahirkheli, N.N., Cherry, A.S., Tackett, A.P., McCaffree, M.A., & Gillaspy, S.R. (2014). Postpartum depression on the neonatal intensive care unit: current perspectives. *International Journal of Women's Health, 6*, 975–987.

Thurgood, S., Avery, D.M., Williamson, L. (2009). Postpartum depression (PPD). *American Journal of Clinical Medicine 6* (2): 17–22.

Tronick, E.Z. (1989). Emotions and emotional communication in infants. *American Psychologist 44 (2)*: 112.

Tronick, E., Beeghley, M. (2011). Infants' meaning-making and the development of mental health problems. *American Psychologist, 66*(2), 107–119.

Tsze, L. (2012). The Speculations on Metaphysics, Polity, and Morality, of the Old Philosopher, Lau-Tsze. (J. Chalmers, trans.) London: Trubner & Co. (Original work published 1868.) Nabu Press.

Uvnas-Moberg, K., Kendall-Tackett, K. (2018). The mystery of D-MER: What can hormonal research tell us about dysphoric milk-ejection reflex? *Clinical Lactation, 9*(1): 23–29. doi:10.1891/2158-0782.9.1.23.

Van der Kolk, B., MD. (2015) *The Body Keeps the Score: Brain, Mind, and Body in the Healing of Trauma.* New York: Penguin Books.

van Deursen-Gelderloos, M., & Bakker, E. (2015). Is EMDR effective for women with posttraumatic stress symptoms after childbirth? *European Health Psychologist, 17*(S), 873.

VanderKruik, R., Barreix, M., Chou, D., Allen, T., Say, L., & Cohen, L.S. (2017). The global prevalence of postpartum psychosis: a systematic review. *BMC Psychiatry, 17:* 272.

Wenzel, A., Haugen, E., Jackson, L., & Robinson, K. (2003). Prevalence of generalized anxiety at eight weeks postpartum. *Archives of Women's Mental Health 6*(1), 43–49.

Wenzel, A. & Kleiman, K. (2014). *Cognitive Behavioral Therapy for Perinatal Distress.* New York: Routledge.

Wharton, E. (1911). *Ethan Frome.* New York: Scribner's.

Wickramaratne, P.J., Weissman, M.N. (1998). Onset of psychopathology in offspring by developmental phase and parental depression. *J Am Acad Child Adolesc Psychiatry, 37:* 933–942.

Wilde, O. (1997). *An Ideal Husband.* London: Methuen & Co. Ltd. (Original published 1893.) Retrieved from Project Gutenberg: www.gutenberg.org/files/885/885-h/885-h.htm

Winnicott, D.W. (1971). *Playing and Reality.* New York: Psychology Press.

Wisner, K.L., Perel, J.M., Peindl, K.S., Hanusa, B.H. (2004). Timing of depression recurrence in the first year after birth. *J Affect Disord,78:* 249–52.

Wisner, K., Sit, D., McShea, M., Rizzo, D., Zoretich, R. Hughes, C., Eng, H., Wisniewski, S., Costantino, M., Confer, A., Moses-Kolko, E., Famy, C., & Hanusa, B. (2013). Onset timing, thoughts of self-harm, and diagnoses in postpartum women with screen-positive depression findings. *JAMA Psychiatry, 70* (5): 490–498.

Woolhouse, H., Gartland, D., Mensah, F., & Brown, S.J. (2015). Maternal depression from early pregnancy to 4 years postpartum in a prospective pregnancy cohort study: implications for primary health care. *BJOG: an international journal of obstetrics and gynaecology, 122*(3): 312–321. https://doi.org/10.1111/1471-0528.12837

Yim, I.S., Stapleton, L.R., & Schetter, C.D. (2015). Biological and psychosocial predictors of postpartum depression: systematic review and call for integration. *Annual Review of Clinical Psychology, 11,* 99–137.

Zambaldi, C.F., Cantilino, A., Montenegro, A.C., Paes, J.A., de Albuquerque, T.L., Sougey, E.B. (2009). Postpartum obsessive-compulsive disorder: prevalence and clinical characteristics. *Compr Psychiatry, 50*(6): 503–509. doi: 10.1016/j.comppsych.2008.11.014.

# INDEX